Forget Memory

Forget Memory

Creating Better Lives for People with Dementia

ANNE DAVIS BASTING

The Johns Hopkins University Press
Baltimore

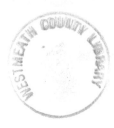
The Johns Hopkins University Press
2715 North Charles Street
Baltimore, Maryland 21218-4363
www.press.jhu.edu

Library of Congress Cataloging-in-Publication Data

Basting, Anne Davis, 1965–
    Forget memory : creating better lives for people with dementia / Anne Davis
Basting.
        p. ; cm.
    Includes bibliographical references and index.
    ISBN-13: 978-0-8018-9249-3 (hardcover : alk. paper)
    ISBN-10: 0-8018-9249-X (hardcover : alk. paper)
    ISBN-13: 978-0-8018-9250-9 (pbk. : alk. paper)
    ISBN-10: 0-8018-9250-3 (pbk. : alk. paper)
    1. Dementia. 2. Memory disorders in old age. I. Title.
    [DNLM: 1. Dementia—psychology—Personal Narratives.   2. Quality of
Life—Personal Narratives. WT 155 B326f 2009]
    RC521.B376 2009
    616.8'3—dc22   2008037842

A catalog record for this book is available from the British Library.

*Special discounts are available for bulk purchases of this book. For more information,
please contact Special Sales at 410-516-6936 or specialsales@press.jhu.edu.*

The Johns Hopkins University Press uses environmentally friendly book
materials, including recycled text paper that is composed of at least 30 percent
post-consumer waste, whenever possible. All of our book papers are acid-free, and
our jackets and covers are printed on paper with recycled content.

To my memory—

Brad, Ben, Will, Tom, Sally, Ellen, Tom Jr., Seth, Susan, Alice, Abe, Alice, Arthur, Grace, Bob, Jane, Eric, Mark, Brenda, Harriet, David, Ken, Katherine, Elinor, Trey, Art, Kelly, Jay, Kathy, Susan, John, Rick, Tom C., Gülgün, David, Kate, Tim, Skip, Eric, Diane, Jim, Judy, Mark, Manya, Howard, Stacy, Jasmine, Aims

and so many more

Contents

Preface

The ideas and stories you'll encounter in these pages emerged from my experiences over the last 15 years working in the fields of the arts and aging. During these years, I have been an artist, a teacher, a writer, and the director of a center on aging. I hope that the stories and thoughts collected here are of use to the broad range of people with whom I've worked. My ideal reader is anyone invested in improving the lives of people with dementia—from health care professionals and those studying to become health care professionals, to families and friends of people with dementia, to people with dementia themselves.

My heartfelt thanks go out to all those who shared the thoughts and experiences that form the substance of much of this book. I want to thank a few in particular whom I might not quote directly in these pages but whose support has given me the courage to think outside the box.

Kathleen Woodward. Kathy's advice, support, and thought-provoking questions have kept me from falling between the academic cracks. *Susan McFadden.* I treasure our lunches at a little family restaurant in Lomira, Wisconsin, exactly halfway between our homes in Appleton and Milwaukee. *Peter Whitehouse.* Over lunches at anonymous restaurants in anonymous conference hotels, Peter and I tumble into conversations that blend medicine, media, art, history. *Stephen Katz.* He's not just a sociologist of aging; he's also a jazz drummer and plays in a rock-and-roll cover band. *Rhonda Montgomery.* When we both happen to be in the office, we catch a few precious minutes together to talk about our latest ideas. I'm thankful for the savvy model she's provided of how to make the system work for me. *Robin Mayrl and all those at the Helen Bader Foundation.* This family foundation and their dedicated program officers supported me when all I had was an idea and some passion. I can't thank them enough for the risks they take in supporting some of the edgiest work in dementia care. When the foundation sunsets, it'll leave an amazing legacy in the field of aging. *Beth Meyer Arnold.* Her vision and courage to try ideas outside her expertise are a daily inspiration. *Jed Levine.* He's one of the people who just gets why the arts work. *Jim Herrington.* He has photographed the Rolling Stones, Cormac McCarthy, and Roger and Rocille McConnell. The field of aging is lucky to have him. *Rick Moody.* He presses the acceleration pedal on any idea. *Tom Fritsch.* His patience and insightful readings of draft versions of this book made it all possible. *Roger and Rocille McConnell.* I'm deeply grateful for their trust and inspiration. And, finally, a heartfelt thanks to all my partners, philanthropic, academic, and community based, who are open to my crazy ideas. *Wendy Harris.* Thank you for helping make it all happen with such grace.

Forget Memory

Introduction

Dementia Is Hard, but It Needn't Be
This Hard

Roger and Rocille McConnell sat uncomfortably in the doctor's office. They knew something was wrong with Roger. They were afraid to hear it named, but they wanted an answer—and to know if there was something they could do about it. They are *doing* kind of people. Roger is an active member of county committees, and Rocille is deeply involved in her synagogue's efforts to promote social justice. So they made the appointment and opened themselves to bad news. Theirs was not an ideal encounter with the medical establishment. "I was not happy . . . because after he told us," says Rocille with a clear edge of anger in her voice, "the psychiatrist walked out. He said, 'My nurse will bring you a packet.' Well, the next day I told him how I felt. I said, 'I can't believe you people deal this way.'" Roger tumbled into depression.

Alice lives in a nursing home. She has little awareness of the last 50 years of her life. When her husband, Bob, visits, she recognizes him as someone she cares for. But when Bob steps back into the elevator, he is wiped clean from her consciousness. For years, Alice and Bob took long walks together. In the nursing home, Alice finds a new friend, a man who walks with her down the hallways, often arm in arm. One day, when Bob visits, he sees Alice and her walking companion strolling down the hall together and becomes irate. "I can't believe you allowed this to happen!" he yells at the staff, insisting that they separate them. Staff members put a care plan into effect to keep the two apart, and Alice's spirits clearly suffer.

Gil cares for Victoria at home. He talks glowingly of their long life together, of raising children, bowling in leagues, ballroom dancing, and going to movies. They were a couple rich with friends. Even with Vic deep in dementia, they dance around the living room when Lawrence Welk comes on the television. Only now, Gil and Vic are alone. Their friends stopped visiting years ago. Gil says he can understand it, can

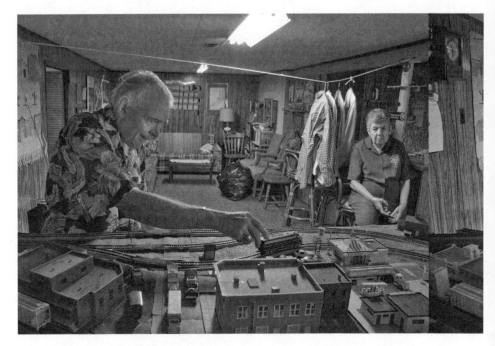

Roger and Rocille McConnell, 2006. Photo by www.jimherrington.com.

understand that people feel awkward around them. But the depth of his loneliness is palpable. He lies awake at night thinking about it.

On an individual level, the physical and psychological challenges of dementia can knock the wind out of you. Whether the diagnosis is yours, your spouse's, your friend's, or your parent's, when dementia comes into your life it can seem to deprive you of every last ounce of your strength. On a societal level, the financial and practical challenges of providing care for someone with an illness that can last up to 15 years may well leave us with few resources to pay for anything else. Certainly, the stories we read about dementia in newspapers, books, and magazines and that we hear about in films and on television and radio ring the alarm, pointing to the catastrophe that will strike when the members of the baby boom generation reach their mid-80s. It is possible that dementia might affect more than half of them—estimates of the numbers of people who will develop dementia by 2050 range from 11 to 16 million.

This book emerges from a single basic question: to what extent do our

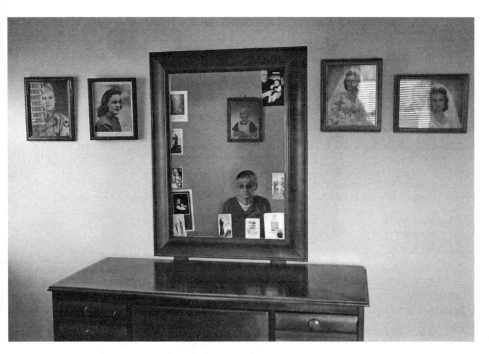

Victoria, 2007. Photo by Wing Young Huie.

fears about dementia and aging contribute to the tragic conditions of living with dementia and the catastrophic economic story of dementia? We all eagerly await a "cure"—if such a thing is possible. We can perhaps more safely place our hopes and research dollars in scientifically informed paths to prevention. But there is another tool we can use to improve the lives of people with dementia and all those who care for them. It is something we can use *now*, while the scientists work on paths to prevention. We can change our *attitudes* and our *care practices*. We can work to reduce the paralyzing stigma and fear that wrap themselves around dementia and Alzheimer's disease, the most prominent form of dementia.

Dementia has always been and probably always will be a frightening experience. But it can also be much more. I was a playwright and first-year PhD student when I began volunteering with people with dementia in 1990. And in the years since then, I have seen people with dementia and people who love them alike nearly drowning in fear, grief, anxiety, and anger. And yet, I've also seen much more. I've seen both people with dementia as well as those who care for them move through their fears and come to feel fierce pride and overwhelmingly joy, to show compassion and selflessness, and to express bawdy humor and dry wit. I hold out hope that sharing stories of people who succeed in moving through fear and learn to live with stigma, who find meaning in the experience of dementia, might help inspire more people to do the same— to see dementia as more than a death sentence. Would that doctor have treated Roger and Rocille the way he did if he had come to terms with his own fears of and discomfort with people with dementia? Would Bob have forbade Alice to walk the halls with her companion if he had more fully understood and accepted Alice's world? Would Gil and Vic be subject to such paralyzing loneliness if their friends had a better grasp of dementia?

We fear dementia. Some of that is natural. Human beings have an innate fear of death that serves us well by making us cautious. Famed neurologist, psychiatrist, and Holocaust survivor Viktor Frankl suggests that we also have an innate fear of meaninglessness. Because a diagnosis of dementia triggers thoughts of both, we avoid thinking about it. We delay seeking diagnosis for ourselves or for our loved ones. We slowly stop visiting friends who are experiencing it. We don't want to think about it, so we satisfy ourselves with a thin layer of general information. A 2006 poll by Harris Interactive showed that while 93 percent of the people they polled had heard of Alzheimer's disease, 74 percent said they knew little or nothing about it.

But ultimately, the fear reflex is making the experience of dementia worse. We are living in the time of dementia. As we live longer than ever before, dementia touches the lives of more of us than ever before. This book aims to burrow into that fear, to directly confront it and thereby come to understand it more fully so that it won't interfere with living a full life with dementia or fully living with and loving people with dementia. By coming to know about and make use of services that might help them, people will be better able to work through their fears and alleviate the tragic social conditions of the disease—the isolation, the stress, the depression. The hope is that doctors will develop a better understanding of the complexity of the dementia experience and so never again say, "My nurse will bring you a packet." That spouses will come to work through their grief in support groups so Alice can still walk down the hallway and feel supported by her new friend. That people will learn not to feel awkward around loved ones with dementia so Gil and Vic do not have to dance alone.

How can we get to such a place? To a world in which the flash of heat that rises from deep within us when we forget where we put the keys for the third time in a week doesn't keep us from being fully present in the company of our neighbor with dementia? A world in which our fears of dementia don't stop nursing, medical, and social work students from studying how to work with people with dementia? A place in which daughters and sons, granddaughters and grandsons, might look forward to spending time with their parent or grandparent with dementia?

Part 1 looks at the root of our fears about dementia. How are people describing their fears? Exactly what is it that people afraid of? Chapter 1 endeavors to address fears of memory loss by clearing up misunderstandings of how memory works. Cultural pressures to remember have given us unrealistic expectations as to how memory should work. We are taxing our memories to the limit at a time when we are living longer than ever. The anxiety over our overworked memories is spilling over, leading us to fear and stigmatize dementia. Chapter 2 dives deeper into just how bias—born of fear, stereotypes, and stigma—might affect those experiencing dementia.

Part 2, chapters 3 through 7, looks at popular culture to see what stories about dementia we're hearing and asks whether those stories capture the complexity of the dementia experience or simply add fuel to our fears. Part 3, chapters 8 through 17, offers brief, alternative stories of dementia, stories in which people are moving through fears of dementia to find meaning within the disease experience. Each of these chapters focuses on a different approach to connecting and communicating when rational language breaks down. These range from dance to painting, from songwriting to the art of conversation. I hope that these 10 unique approaches might provide models for people struggling to find a way to be in the company of loved ones experiencing dementia—or for readers with dementia struggling to find a way to express themselves to others.

Finally, the conclusion outlines some concrete steps for changing attitudes toward and care practices of people with dementia on a national scale. Just what we can do to improve the lives of people with dementia today? We all wait for a pill that will ensure that no matter how long we live, we will have the ability to live meaningful lives surrounded by people who care about us. But while we wait for the scientific discoveries, there is a great deal we can do right now to enrich ourselves and the lives of others. We can only do so, however, if we learn to respond to people with dementia with more than just fear.

Just what is it that we are afraid of? I asked the question of more than 30 people: doctors, family care partners, people with dementia, and college students who had barely heard the term. What did they say?

Part One

UNDERSTANDING OUR FEARS ABOUT DEMENTIA

➤ This is why I call this a time capsule. . . . If someone digs it up in the future, they are bound to say: look at what they didn't know. Look at what they failed to understand. Look at these curious creatures. Why were they so afraid?

Michael Ignatieff

To better understand the roots of our fears about dementia, I led a team of researchers through a series of interviews with people with dementia, people who have friends or parents with dementia, and professionals (doctors, nurses, social workers) who work in dementia care. How did these folks explain their fears? And what seems to be underneath them?

Fear of Being a Burden

By far, the fear of being a burden was the most common response. We hear this a lot, but what exactly does it mean? Joan is an energetic, middle-aged woman with two college-aged daughters. When asked what scares her about dementia, she quickly pinpoints "being a burden": "I especially fear being a burden to other people. Because it's just not the way I have ever seen myself. I'm a very independent person, and I like doing things for myself. I'm used to being the mom and the wife and the person who takes care of everything for everybody else. That's my role in life. That's who I am. And to lose that would be to lose myself, lose my identity. And that terrifies me."

Mary, whose mother is experiencing increasing troubles with her memory, said much the same thing: "Generally, I don't think anyone looks forward to getting old and being dependent. I mean, we're all going to die of something. . . . You just want it to be quick and not a burden."

Billy, whose mother also had dementia, was even less subtle. "I hope I die in my sleep," he said. "I hope not to be a burden to anyone."

The people we interviewed described a fierce pride in being "independent" and in enabling their children, friends, and spouses to live full, independent lives. In their view, if you had dementia, you were emotionally, physically, and financially enslaving those you love to your care. They saw shame in such "dependency." No one described the experience of dementia as positive in any way, for either the person going through it or the family members. No one imagined the caregiving experience had the potential to be reciprocal. Instead, all the responses about being a burden assumed that the person with dementia takes while the caregiver gives and gives and gives.

Fear of the Unknown

Marilyn, who works as an aide in a nursing home, talked of her fears in terms of the randomness of who dementia strikes. "It's sad to me," says Marilyn in soft tones. "It hurts my feelings. It makes you feel that one day, I could wake up and it could be me, it could be one of my loved ones. Your body is a mystery, and I guess we will never truly understand how the body really works." Rocille worded it slightly differently: "My biggest fear is the unknown. No one is able to predict how long Roger will be able to function to the point that I don't need to be with him 24/7. When that time comes, I will lose my best friend and partner. We have such a loving, caring, wonderful relationship and life, and I dread when that vanishes."

Darren, who works as an aide in a long-term care setting, brought up another component to fearing the unknown—that people experiencing dementia can look at a face or object and not know who or what it is. In dementia, what is unknown encompasses not just the future ("What will happen tomorrow?") but the present ("What is that thing? Why am I feeling this way?"). "We take a lot of things for granted in life," said Darren, "something as simple as waking up and knowing where the bathroom is. Knowing where the car is, where to get breakfast. I think the biggest fear is of the unknown." This particularly frightened Darren when he thought about his young family. Forgetting the faces of his wife and children seemed incomprehensible to him.

The "not knowing" of dementia can drive us to distraction. Will I get it? Will it get worse? How much worse? When? The shifting sands of medical research and advice, the uniqueness of each pathway through the dementia experience, and the creep of the unknown into the people, objects, and feelings we take for granted are clearly at the root of our fears of getting it or watching a loved one move through it.

Fear of Being Out of Control

For Billy's mother, dementia was, in some ways, a blessing. She had always been a difficult and bitter person, wounded by years of little betrayals. Dementia eased her anger, and Billy found he enjoyed her company more after the illness than before. But he was still haunted. "She didn't seem to be in control of herself," he said. The dementia experience seems to sever a person from his or her intentions.

"That's not him, it's the disease," we say, when a man with dementia shouts out in anger. "That's not her, that's the disease," we say if a woman with dementia peppers her conversation with vulgarities. Separating the person from the actions can help us cope with some significant personality changes in ourselves and those we love. But staff members of a nursing home might also say, "That's not him, that's the dementia" if a man cries out in pain and asks for help. Or insists on waffles instead of pancakes. Or asks to call his son. "It's the disease" severs intentionality from both unusual behavior and everyday actions alike.

We fear this global dismissal of intention and the subsequent inability to affect the course of our day-to-day lives. Those with dementia may lose control over their lives no matter where they live, but it is more likely to happen in a facility setting. Even though it *shouldn't*, institutional living can mean sacrificing your autonomy for the ease of the system that is attending to your physical needs. For example, you might be able to go to the bathroom with the help of an attendant, but when that attendant has eight people to get up and dressed, chances are good that you'll be in diapers. People we interviewed likened living without choice, without autonomy, to "not really living."

The experience of dementia can also mean the loss of simple freedoms that give us a certain dominion over our lives. Like a driver's license. In the United States, where daily life is organized around the automobile, losing the ability to drive can seem catastrophic. Suddenly, someone who has been able to get to doctor appointments, the grocery store, pharmacy, senior center, and friends' houses must endlessly ask and wait for rides. Or stay home. Simply crossing a parking lot to get from one big box store to another can be impossible for older adults with physical and cognitive disabilities. A survey of 335 older adults showed that the fear of losing their driver's license was a key reason they put off seeing a doctor about their memory loss.

Fear of Being Violated or Robbed

"It saddens my heart that you could be robbed of something that you had worked for all of your life," said Marilyn. We have come to see our memories as things that we have, collect, and build on to create a unique sense of self. When someone begins to lose access to memories, it can feel as though something that is rightfully his or hers is being unfairly taken away. On a more practical level, caring for someone with dementia in our broken health care system can mean financial impoverishment not just for individuals but for entire families. It's easy to feel "robbed." The people we interviewed expressed both anger and fear over working hard to plan and save, only to have it all go toward the costs of dementia care, which can go on for many years. Spending one's savings on dementia care can be especially painful because *good* care is so hard to find. In that same survey of 335 adults, 40 percent said they feared that a diagnosis of dementia would mean losing their insurance—something that would lead to impoverishment or, at the very least, poor care options.

Fear of a Meaningless Existence

"He who has a *why* to live for can bear with almost any *how*," wrote philosopher Friedrich Nietzsche in 1895. Viktor Frankl includes this quotation in *Man's Search for Meaning,* his 1946 eyewitness account of how a sense of purpose and faith in the future enabled people to survive the horror of the concentration camps. The people we interviewed described dementia, particularly the end stages, as void of meaning. One of the young people put it this way: "I feel it [Alzheimer's] is possibly the worst thing that could happen to a person given . . . the way our society is, at least, the Western society. Everything is about being productive members of society, about being active with friends and family, your church, everything. The brain is what makes [people] go and enjoy things in life. It's all because of memory." If you lose your memory, his logic flowed, "it's probably really, really frustrating." In the survey of 335 older adults, 50 percent said they feared becoming depressed and 45 percent feared becoming anxious. With cultural attitudes that tell us that caregivers *give* and people with dementia *take,* endlessly and pointlessly, their fears are well founded.

Scientists are working hard to discover how dementia works, who gets it, why, and what might stop it. They are working to identify people with memory problems earlier and earlier in the hope of following them through the disease process and seeing what kinds of treatment are most effective. This work must continue. But these core fears—of being a burden, of being out of control, of being violated or robbed, and of a meaningless existence—can be eased by changes in attitude, awareness, and care practices and policies. I don't pretend that we can eliminate the fear of dementia. We are human, after all. We can, though, learn to feel *more* than fear. We can learn to feel and act with respect and compassion and to believe in purpose for those with dementia and those who love and care for them.

To work through fear and confront head on its companions, stigma, denial, and stereotype, we first need to better understand the nature of memory. What can and should we expect of memory? How did we come to view memory as the center of our identity?

What Is (and Isn't) Memory?

How a Better Understanding of Memory
Might Ease Our Fears about Its Loss

> ❧ But what I am getting at is that re-membering is essentially not only
> an act of retrieval, but a creative thing, it happens in the moment;
> it's an act, an act . . . of the imagination.
>
> *Mnemonic*

Memory loss is just one of the symptoms of dementia, but it is the one
that most grabs our attention, particularly in the early stages. When the
face of someone at a party offers no clues to a name or when we stand,
blank faced, in a parking lot with no idea where we left the car, worry
rushes through us.

What can we expect of memory? What's normal? Are some of our
fears based on unrealistic ideas of what memory is capable of? The
boundary between normal memory loss and dementia, particularly in
the early stages, can be blurry. How we understand and how we value
memory can contribute to our fear of its loss. Contemporary American
culture puts great pressure on us to remember that exacerbates our fears
of memory loss. My aim here is to alleviate some of that pressure by putting memory into historical context. And, because I believe that memory is story, I pepper tales of my own throughout the chapter by way of
example.

Memory is how we store and retrieve our experiences, from the
mundane to the profound. When we retrieve memory, we create story.
We come to understand ourselves, others, and the world around us by
listening to and telling stories. This process of storing and retrieving
and retelling experiences enables us to respond to new experiences,
apply what we know, and learn and grow from such encounters. It enables us to track our experiences across time, form a narrative about
what those experiences mean, and create a sense of "self" in time, based
on that narrative.

I have memories of playing elaborate, solitary imagination games when I was a kid. In "wild animal veterinarian," for example, I would boldly push through two honeysuckle bushes in the long line of them that bordered our house and a neighboring field and imagine I was entering the savannah to tend to a sick zebra. Enter between two other bushes, and voila, a wounded elephant that urgently needed my attention. In college, I found my passion in Jim Yaffe's creative writing class, held around a table in the second floor of a white clapboard house. In graduate school and beyond, I let my imagination fly out my fingers click-clacking on the computer keyboard. Out of those separate memories, I build a story of self—that of a writer. In turn, I ask, "What's your story?" (perhaps not so overtly) as a way to understand and relate to other people. Memory is story, and storytelling is the process through which we know and grow ourselves and our communities, small and large.

We attempt to understand memory in many ways. We study memory on a molecular level through neuroscience research. We seek to grasp how the mind functions through cognitive psychology. We explore ways to make memory more efficient by inventing "external" memories like computers, palm pilots, or something as simple as post-it notes. We look at social and historical trends in the valuation, facilitation, and shaping of memory in different places and times. We study memory by representing—telling stories about—what it feels like to experience it or to lose it.

We have ample proof that memory has fascinated humankind since the days of the early Greeks. That fascination has not only persisted but is today raging. In the last 25 years, writing and research about and representation of memory has surged. The United States is obsessed with memory. Perhaps this is because, as a young country, we have so little of it. Or perhaps because as a country of immigrants that was built largely through the destruction of native cultures and on the backs of people stolen from their homes, we have a lot of memories to reassemble. A century of world wars and genocide that threatened to destroy the collective memory of entire cultures has also launched multiple imperatives to remember as a way to heal and guard against horrors of such magnitude happening again. Certainly, technological advances have fueled the study of memory. Collaborations among biologists, neurologists, and cognitive psychologists, spurred on by the development of imaging techniques that enable us to see activity in the brain (PET, MRI, CT, etc.), have pushed our understanding of memory to new levels. This burst of memory research across the disciplines has helped paint a new picture of what memory is and isn't.

So, just what is and isn't memory? And how do our cultural views about memory contribute to our attitudes and fears about dementia?

A Single Memory Is Not Encoded into a Single Nerve Cell

On the molecular level, we now know, memories are stored and transmitted through nerve cells, and different parts of the brain support different components of a given memory. My friend Gülgün makes a shepherd's pie that, try as I might, I cannot replicate. My memory of her making shepherd's pie includes the smell of browning turkey sausage; the colors of the carrots and peas; my emotional response (which is weak-kneed envy and gratitude); my understanding of the physical procedures (even though it doesn't taste the same when I prepare it); and, above all, the taste. These elements of my memory of Gülgün's shepherd's pie are not all encoded into one nerve cell but dispersed in various parts of the brain.

There Is Not Just One Kind of Memory

Memory takes many different forms. There is "long-term memory," which is memory of events in the past. "Short-term memory" is of events that occurred recently (in approximately the last 18 seconds). "Working memory" is the shortest of all; it encompasses the details and numbers we keep for only a few seconds until our brains decide they won't need them anymore. We also have "episodic memory" (specific events, people, and information), "semantic memory" (relating to general knowledge), and "procedural memory" (relating to how we do things). "I gave you an apple yesterday" is an episodic memory, while "apples are red" is a semantic memory. Knowing what to do with an apple one is holding (eat it, in most contexts) is procedural memory. Finally, we have "implicit memory" (or subconscious memory) and "explicit memory" (conscious). Each one of these types of memory is stored in a different way and in a different place in the brain, so different disease processes affect them in unique ways. The result is that some people in the advanced stages of Alzheimer's disease, for example, can demonstrate learning through implicit and semantic memory even when their explicit and/or episodic memory is severely limited.

What We Remember Is a Balance of Outside and Inside Influences

"There is no point," writes Maurice Halbwachs, "in seeking where [memories] are preserved in my brain or in some nook of my mind to which I alone have access: for they are recalled by me externally, and the groups of which I am a part at any time give me the means to reconstruct them." My maternal grandmother was a strong influence on my life, and I tell many stories about her. She taught me to ride horses, to make a bed with hospital corners, and to love both the *McNeil-Lehrer* news show and Omar Sharif in *Dr. Zhivago*. But I notice that when I'm talking with strangers, the stories I tell about Grandma Cantwell are quite different from the ones I tell when I'm in the presence of my mother or my cousin—both of whom experienced a different version of my grandmother, who could be, well, not so nice. In fact, she had a healthy mean streak. I want to be sensitive to their experiences, so I remember Grandma slightly differently when I'm with them. I tell stories that fit their memories of her. Like the one about how after she died, the family found a small box with a hand-scrawled note that said, "Congratulations, you found my gold!" It contained her gold-filled molars. That first time I rode horses with Grandma, the encoded memories physically changed my brain. But every time I recall that story—of how I ended up in a pile of manure after she "encouraged" the horse to rear up and then dared me to get back on—I create a new memory that also physically changes my brain. And thus, the biological and social components of memory cannot be separated.

Similarly, I sometimes feel like I never went to college. I find it tough to remember specific events during my 4 years there, which were, on the whole, quite fulfilling. But when I went back to Colorado Springs for my twentieth college reunion in 2007, and my eyes traced the landscape of red rocks and gnarled pines against the backdrop of Pike's Peak, I was suddenly flooded with specific names, faces, and moments I had no idea that I had retained.

My mother tells a story that demonstrates another way in which memory is a social process. Every year a friend of the family would give us an amazing cheesecake for Christmas. Every year my mother asked for the recipe so we wouldn't have to wait another 12 months to taste it, and every year he said no. Out of desperation (she has a serious sweet tooth), my mother told him a story about two elderly sisters, both ex-

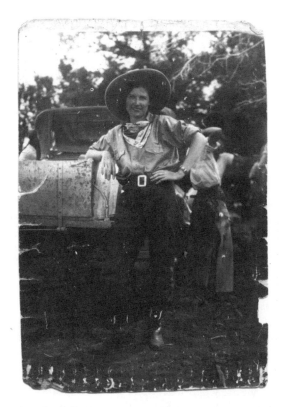

My grandmother Alice Davis Cantwell. Photographer unknown.

cellent cooks. Every time one of the sisters brought food to a sick friend or a new mother in their neighborhood, she'd slip in a meticulously printed copy of the recipe. The other sister was equally generous with her cooking but never included the recipes. She preferred to be needed. Then, through an unfortunate act of fate, their house caught fire. They lost everything. With the help of friends, the sisters set up house in a new apartment. Slowly, their new home filled with food, and attached to each pot or pan were the recipes that the one sister had so carefully written out. The other sister's recipes, however, disappeared in the fire.

I could tell the same story about backing up my computer more often, but you get the point. And so did our friend, who promptly gave us the cheesecake recipe. And I remember him fondly every time I see that sour cream topping crack golden brown. We rely on external memory aids—other human beings, objects, or the landscape—to process

and remember things we cannot successfully store and retrieve ourselves. Memory and story, and the selves we build with them, are crafted
in relationship to the world around us—the people, the places, and the
cultural influences. The world around us significantly influences how
we encode our experiences, how (and if) we retrieve them, and how we
make meaning of them. Memory is, in other words, a relational process.

Memory Is Not a Camera Aimed at the Past

In some ways, technology has provided us with misleading metaphors
for memory. Thanks to the computer, the camera, and the museum, we
have a tendency to think of a memory as a bit of information that is
stored away and can be retrieved on demand, as a photograph or video
that objectively captures all details of a moment, or as an artifact that,
with the right care, will remain intact for centuries. But in reality, a
memory is none of these things. When information is encoded, it does
create a physical change in the brain. But we filter retrieved memories
through who we have become and all the subsequent experiences we've
had since the moment that piece of information entered our minds. A
memory is not an object preserved in the museum of our minds. It is a
living, changeable thing that is shaped by who we are when we encode
it and by who we are when we retrieve it. For example, I remember the
game of "wild animal veterinarian" differently now, with a lens of 42
years, from when I was 15.

Some Memory Loss Is Normal, Even Necessary

No one's memory is perfect. Stories of those who have nearly perfect recall ("S" in A. R. Luria's *Mind of a Mnemonist,* for example, could remember extensive, random strings of numbers years after he'd read
them) also describe these folks as being unable to function normally in
society. Because our minds must process so much of our daily lives, our
brains make calculated bets. They filter out what is not likely to be important to us later and retain what is. In *The Seven Sins of Memory: How
the Mind Forgets and Remembers,* Daniel Schacter points out the following categories describing how human memory fails us. *Transience* is the
weakening of our memory over time and is to blame for the majority of
our memory problems. *Absent mindedness* keeps us from paying enough

attention to something to enable it to be properly encoded in our memory. In this case, it's not that I forget where I put my keys. It's that I was so distracted by talking on my cell phone that I never put the information into my memory. *Blocking* refers to being unable to retrieve a specific piece of information. Transience, absent mindedness, and blocking are all "sins" of omission. Schacter's remaining four are sins of commission in which the information is present, but as he writes, it is either "incorrect or unwanted." These four "sins" include *misattribution,* in which we assign a memory to the wrong source; *suggestibility,* in which a memory is implanted by someone else; *bias,* in which current beliefs influence how we retrieve a memory; and *persistence,* in which a disturbing memory seems to haunt us. He argues, however, that these "sins" are not a fall from a state of memory perfection. Instead, their purpose is to keep us from remembering everything—and, in the process, getting hopelessly lost in the details of life. A certain amount of forgetting is a necessary and positive feature of our humanity.

Some age-related memory loss is normal. "It would actually be quite abnormal for someone *not* to have increasing memory challenges in their seventies, eighties, and beyond," writes Peter Whitehouse. Still, even if it is normal, that might not stop us from trying to conquer it. Normal, age-related memory loss could become the new wrinkles. Botox, skin creams, and cosmetic surgery sprung up around our disdain for normal, aging skin, and now it seems the cognitive equivalent of calisthenics is being touted as is the way to eliminate or hide normal, age-related memory loss.

Memory Has a History

I counted no fewer than 20 books written in the last 5 years that offer to improve your memory. Gaming companies have also discovered the "memory" market. "Give your brain the workout it needs" reads the advertising for Brain Age and Brain Age2, the new "brain trainer" by Nintendo. According to Schacter, the theories on which these books rely are largely the same as those that informed the visual mnemonics (or memory systems) of the early Greeks and inventions like Camillo's Memory Theatre in late medieval Italy. Simply put, the more we associate our experiences with stories and images, the better we'll be able to encode and retrieve them. "S" in Luria's *Mind of a Mnemonist* created elaborate visualizations of stories that enabled him to recall those long lists of random numbers, sometimes years later. But what *has* changed between Greek epic poems (recited from memory) and today's Blackberries?

Historians have dedicated entire careers to tackling small pieces of the great puzzle of memory and its partner, forgetting. No single book can answer the multitude of questions that memory raises. How is memory valued? How is memory practiced? How is memory understood? And each of these questions also begs to be answered for every cultural moment and every cultural context. I find French historian Jacques Le Goff's ideas helpful as an overarching framework (even though he looks at only Western culture, he aims his lens primarily on the fields of history and anthropology, and his view of the earliest forms of memory seems a little romantic). Le Goff identifies five major shifts in how memory has been perceived during the course of Western culture. In the first phase, which occurred before written language, memory was creative, vital, free flowing, and alive. Exalted elders were charged with being the memory of their tribes, groups, or families. In the absence of externalizing devices (like the written word), memory existed in people's minds and between them, and it was transposed onto nature through ritual and spoken stories. Since there was no written form of language at the time, we don't know much about this time period. It is likely, however, that their ideas did filter down to those who could capture them on paper.

Le Goff's second phase was initiated with the development of written language and the externalization of memory—that is, the storing or recording it outside of our minds and spoken words. Writing brought with it the ability to inscribe meaning onto monuments. In this time period, a king now had more control over how the story of a particular battle or of his life was told. Libraries, archives, and museums began to emerge as repositories for safeguarding the stories of urban, royal life. In Greek culture, memory entered the realm of the divine in the form of the goddess Mnemosyne (Memory), the mother of the nine muses conceived in nine nights spent with Zeus. As Greek philosophers wrestled with the secular meaning of memory, the myth of Mnemosyne tapped into the human longing for immortality. To drink of the river Lethe, fed by the springs of Oblivion, was to forget all earthly knowledge—of pain and pleasure alike. But to drink of the fountain of Memory was to become immortal. While they were still among the living, mortals could improve their memories through "mnemotechnology"—mnemonic aids that enabled the great rhetoricians and poets of the day to speak without notes.

Le Goff's third phase developed during the medieval period, in which memory, particularly in Western Europe, became "Christianized." He points to the Judeo-Christian roots of concepts of memory and forgetting, in which *forgetting* God's teachings is akin to abandoning God and to being abandoned by God in turn. The medieval period also sees the beginning of the memorializing of the dead, particularly of dead saints. Jewish and Christian communities alike kept *libri memoriales,* in which the stories of important community members were recorded. Much like drinking of the fountain of Memory, being recorded in the *libri memoriales* was a means to becoming immortal, a way to live on in the memory of your community for generations to come. Those who were excommunicated were struck from the book and from the official memory of the community. What I found most intriguing about the medieval period was the flowering of mnemotechnology. Elaborate maps and symbolic systems that Frances Yates so beautifully captures in her 1966 book *The Art of Memory* make our contemporary computer programs and books on improving memory look crass and void of imagination. Yates tells of Camillo's Memory Theater, which was a room purposefully and elaborately arranged with occult images. Supposedly, these images told the story of the history of the universe, and if you coded your personal memories according to these symbols, you could remember your entire life in a single moment.

Le Goff sees the fourth phase as nothing short of a total revolution in memory. During the Renaissance, the advent of the printing press transformed memory by making it more external than it had ever been before. More and more, memory was something you researched, compiled, and archived, not something you held in your mind. After the printing press, one didn't need Camillo's Memory Theater to organize one's mind—one needed an assistant to organize one's filing cabinets and mementos. The sheer volume of information to which regular people (i.e., not priests or kings) had access swelled to an enormous proportion in comparison to what information people could expect to keep in their heads alone. Archives sprang up. The number of memorials, museums, and commemorative events all increased dramatically, suggesting that we needed help to remember what we would otherwise forget. Aristocrats began to write memoirs in the mid-1500s. Dictionaries and encyclopedias were developed to catalog and capture the meaning of words and ideas. A series of revolutions (French, American, Russian) encouraged the opening of the doors of private museums and libraries to the public.

In the twentieth century, Le Goff points to two important developments in how we understand memory. First is what he sees as the pinnacle of honoring the dead—the creation of the Tomb of the Unknown Soldier. This elaborate marking of a nameless individual was meant to bring together a nation through one symbolic act of collective memory. Second is photography. Suddenly, what we could see hazily in our mind's eye, we could now compare to the eye of the camera. Suddenly, memory was visual. Photography has completely revolutionized the way we think about and practice individual and family memory, just as it has radically transformed our expectations of memory. As cameras and film went down in price and photography became more accessible to middle-class families, people came to expect photographs of the significant events of their lives, as well as the everyday moments that would otherwise be filtered out by our mind's selective processes.

The fifth phase Le Goff outlines is our own time period. Today, electronic media create a flood of "data" that we struggle to "manage." Le Goff characterizes technological innovations after 1950 as engendering another radical transformation in memory, and I agree. Computers get smaller and smaller and their chips store more and more memory. What we have the capacity to remember outside of our individual brains now seems endless. What does this ability do to our desire to remember? How does it affect our expectations of individual memory? In my own life I have countless objects that might be considered memory "prosthetics"—computers, journals, photo albums, scrapbooks, flash drives, Palm Pilots, even old-fashioned, hand-drawn calendars that I hang on my refrigerator in a desperate attempt to make sure I am where I need to be when I need to be there. In the last decade, big box stores such as Target and Wal-Mart have added entire aisles dedicated to scrapbooking, enabling young and old alike to creatively select, arrange, and preserve the moments of their lives. A new field has been invented: "personal historians" now have a professional organization to help them market themselves to people who don't want to (or don't feel they can) write the story and gather the artifacts of their own lives. Cameras are a standard feature on our cell phones and can take still or moving pictures that can be instantly emailed to friends or uploaded to YouTube. Retired computer engineer Gordon Bell is hard at work storing his entire life—

everything he sees, everything he does—in a computer program called MyLifeBits that Microsoft hopes will appeal to aging baby boomers. There are now companies that will even make video collages of your life and embed them in your gravestone. Perhaps soon we'll need "quiet zones" in cemeteries like we now need "quiet cars" on trains.

It seems that we now have both the tools and the desire to remember everything. But why? And do we *really* need or want to? Have we come to focus so much on the collection and preservation of the data of our lives that we've lost the ability to live in the moment? The amount of information available and the speed with which is it produced in the early twenty-first century has been the topic of much talk among scholars and writers. Some see it as being accompanied by a decay of "tradition," of the large, mythic stories that used to help us organize ourselves and our individual identities and to establish our purpose and our paths in life. Without these epic stories, the massive flow of information can seem like musical notes without a score—without rhythm or harmony. How can we be expected to order all this information? How can we possibly remember things if they are without form? The Greeks used rhyme and meter to commit their enormous epic poems to memory. Camillo used occult images to organize memories in his Memory Theater. Information is almost impossible for us to retain if it does not form a pattern. Indeed, our period, sometimes called "postmodern," is often described as one in which people are suffering from "social amnesia." Ironically, some have even equated it with the conditions of dementia or schizophrenia.

Over the long sweep of Western history, we have moved from experiencing memory as a vital living thing existing inside of and between us toward thinking of it as something outside of us that we purchase and maintain. Perhaps one thing has stayed the same. Whether we drink of the Greek fountain of Memory, whether we get ourselves written into the medieval *libri memoriales,* or whether we record our lives using Microsoft's MyLifeBits, memory seems to promise us a way out of our shrinking brains and frail bodies and into immortality. As we focus our labor on the act of remembering, both for ourselves and for future generations, we also exacerbate the shame and fear surrounding forgetting and the human frailty, dependency, and mortality with which forgetting is linked.

Memory is nothing if not complex. The "seven sins" of memory enable us to select the most important things to remember from among the flood of information that washes over us in any given moment. We encode and distribute these experiences in multiple ways throughout our brains and bodies. What we select to remember will depend on who we are. Who we are, in turn, is built out of what we have selected to remember. The cultural moment, the environment, and the reasons we want to recall a piece of information all influence how we will arrange and interpret those memories.

The formulas "self = memory" and "loss of memory = loss of self," which inform so much of our thinking about people with dementia and determine how we care for them, seem terribly simplistic once we recognize the intense complexity of memory. Can a memory truly be "lost"? Or is it simply inaccessible? Can a portion of a memory be retrievable while other parts are not? Just how *much* memory loss means a loss of self? And how can we tell? Aren't some kinds of new memories possible for people to encode and access even in late stages of what we call Alzheimer's disease? It seems, given the remaining mysteries and intense complexity of memory, that it would be wise to rigorously examine our obsessions with memory, adjust our expectations, and help people with memory loss better encode, trigger, and express their memories before we declare them lost.

When we look across history, we can see how our society has increasingly put pressure on us to store an ever greater number of memories and to have them at the ready for recall. To more fully understand this pressure to remember and the anxiety that forgetting engenders, I look at specific cultural evidence—the stories we tell about memory loss in the mainstream, in film and on television. What do they tell us about how we value memory? What do they tell us about memory loss? Understanding the stories we tell about memory loss, and how those stories affect us, is the next step on the journey of working through our fears of memory loss and improving the quality of life of those who have dementia and those who care for them.

2

The Danger of Stories

How Stereotypes and the Stigma of Aging and Dementia Can Hurt Us

> ✤ If not turned round when we entered, answered when we spoke, or minded what we did, but if every person we met "cut us dead," and acted as if we were non-existing things, a kind of rage and impotent despair would ere long well up in us, from which the cruelest bodily tortures would be a relief; for these would make us feel that, however bad might be our plight, we had not sunk to such a depth as to be unworthy of attention at all.
>
> William James

Think about the words "memory loss." What images come to mind?

How about "dementia"? "Alzheimer's disease"?

Where do those images come from? Personal experience? The experience of friends? The public image machines of television, film, radio, web, or print media? If you don't have strong, immediate memories of you, your family, or friends going through the experience, it might be hard to think of a source. That's because popular culture belongs to the world of implicit memory. You can't recall it consciously, but it still influences you. You might even adopt it as your own experience. For years I was convinced I had been to the bottom of the Grand Canyon. Then, by happenstance, I caught a glimpse of a rerun of *The Brady Bunch,* and I realized, watching them bouncing down the trail on donkeys, that my memory of my Grand Canyon trip wasn't mine at all. Pop culture is the background noise of our lives. But this begs a bigger question. If pop cultural images of aging and dementia aren't in our conscious memory, do they have any impact on our lives or on the lives of others?

The answer is, "Yes." From the fodder of popular culture, we can form *stereotypes* of older people, which include stereotypes of people with dementia. We apply those stereotypes to others and to ourselves (self-stereotypes). If we hold fast to stereotypes of aging, even when we see evidence to the contrary, we develop a *bias* against older people. If we act on those biases, avoiding older adults, treating them disrespectfully or worse, we are practicing *discrimination*. Bias and discrimination are evidence of *stigma*. In his 1963 book, *Stigma: Notes on the Management of Spoiled Identity*, Erving Goffman takes us back to the early Greek use of the term, which referred to the marks that were cut or burned into the flesh of people to show that they were slaves, criminals, or traitors. In contemporary usage, "stigma" refers to an attribute that deeply discredits a person, marking him or her as thoroughly bad, dangerous, or weak. In Goffman's words, a stigmatized person is "reduced in our minds from a whole and usual person to a tainted, discounted one."

Little research has been done that specifically explores the stigma of and bias against people with dementia. There isn't even a good word to describe the expression of bias against someone with dementia, other than the general term "ageism," the demonstration of bias against older adults. The general categories of "healthism" and "ableism" get some play among people who study disabilities. There are the awkward terms "athazagoraphobia" (fear of forgetting) and "dementophobia" (fear of insanity), but "athazism" and "dementism" don't exactly roll off the tongue. So for now, we must study the bias against people with dementia through two lenses: ageism and the stigma of mental illness.

Compared to racism and sexism, we know little about the roots and mechanics of ageism. Because a fear of and prejudice against older people is still assumed to be normal ("of course, we're afraid of that!" goes the logic), it is wildly understudied. Some theorists explain ageism by suggesting that it has an evolutionary function and that negative feelings about old people are rooted in our primal instincts to avoid death. We do know a few things about ageism. On the whole, people see older adults as "warm" but "incompetent." We like them but find them useless—a sentiment dangerously close to pity. Amy Cuddy, Michael Norton, and Susan Fiske, the researchers who uncovered this demeaning attitude, had hoped that it would be limited to Western cultures, which revere physical appearance and individual independence. But when they studied Asian cultures, in which an individual is more fully knitted into a community or collective identity, they were disappointed to find that even in these more collective cultures, the stereotypes of old people were the same: warm but incompetent. It seems that negative stereotypes about aging accompany globalization—at least among the people who responded to Cuddy, Norton, and Fiske's surveys.

Mary Lou Hummert's work in stereotypes of aging laid the ground-work for the field. In a study published in 1990, Hummert outlines common positive and negative stereotypes of older people held by the young and old alike. On the positive side, stereotypes of aging include the "Golden Ager," the "Perfect Grandparent," the "Activist," the "Small-Town Neighbor," and the "John Wayne Conservative." On the negative side, stereotypes of aging ranged from the "Shrew/Curmudgeon" and the "Elitist" to the "Mildly Impaired," the "Severely Impaired," the "Vulnerable," and the "Despondent" older person. Hummert found that the older the person, the more likely it is that he or she will be seen through the lens of negative stereotypes.

How do older adults themselves describe the experience of ageism? Erdman Palmore, who has done extensive research on aging and stereotypes, found that when he polled older adults, they reported that incidents of ageism are widespread and frequent in their lives. Palmore's surveys show that ageism manifests itself in disrespect or the assumption that older people are disabled in some way by their age (that they have, for example, hearing loss or dementia).

Clearly, negative stereotypes about aging are resulting in bias and discrimination. And how does the stigma of age and dementia affect those confronted with it? For one thing, it might shorten their lives. A study by Becca Levy, Stanislaw Fasl, and Suzanne Kunkel found that negative self-images about aging among elderly people were associated with an average loss of 7.5 years from their life expectancy. The research team seemed shocked by these results. In the conclusion of their article, the researchers suggest that if this loss of 7.5 years was due to a virus, there would be major research dollars fueling a high-stakes search for a cure. But because negative attitudes about aging are assumed to be "normal," we seem resigned to give up 7.5 years of life.

Other studies suggest that a certain amount of cognitive loss might be triggered by the way other people treat you. In a study of people living in nursing homes, a group of older people were given a puzzle and told that, because it was hard, they would receive "help" to complete it. Those who were "helped" with the puzzle had more problems completing it than those who weren't.

In another study, Becca Levy found that people in cultures isolated from negative imagery about aging showed higher cognitive functioning. And in yet another study, Levy and colleagues found that when older adults were exposed to positive images about aging, they performed better on cognitive tests. When older adults were exposed to negative images about aging and cognitive abilities, however, their scores dropped. In the conclusion to this last study, Levy's team toys with two interpretations: "The pessimistic one is that older individuals' memory capabilities can be damaged by self-stereotypes that are derived from a prevalent and insidious stereotype about aging. Specifically, the stereotype that memory decline is inevitable can become a self-fulfilling prophecy." The optimistic reading of the study is that "memory decline is not inevitable." Sticks and stones may break our bones, but names, it seems, can drop our scores on cognitive tests.

This is *not* to say that stereotypes *cause dementia*. The "memory decline" that Levy's research team refers to is not a disease but falls within the realm of "normal" aging. It is clear, however, that stereotypes can influence the way a person experiences both aging and dementia. Age stereotypes can yield patronizing behaviors like speaking in a high perky voice, talking only of simple subjects ("How about that weather!"), using overly simple words in a singsong pitch, giving exaggerated praise ("Oh! That's so *good*, Mr. Miller!"), or ignoring, dismissing, or outright avoiding an older person. People with dementia commonly describe the experience of doctors and nurses talking past them, instead addressing their spouse or care partner. Not surprisingly, residents in long-term care respond to being patronized by withdrawing from activities, and they report having less personal control and less self-esteem.

The stigma surrounding dementia can also keep people from asking about and getting the services that might make their lives better. A 2006 survey sponsored by the Alzheimer's Foundation of America and Forest Pharmaceuticals asked caregivers if and when they took their loved one to be diagnosed. The survey found that typical patients experienced symptoms for just over 2 years before receiving the Alzheimer's diagnosis. In some cases, it was as long as 6 years before a diagnosis was sought. Why the delay? Just over half of all caregivers in the survey (57 percent) mentioned that fear of stigma, including "their own fear of stigma, the patient's fear of stigma, the patient not wanting to see the doctor, and/or the caregiver not wanting to think something could be wrong with their loved one" contributed to the delay in diagnosis. Those caregivers who specifically mention their own and/or their loved one's fear of stigma (14 percent of a total of 539 caregivers interviewed) reported that their loved one waited even longer than the average 2 years for diagnosis. Instead, this group waited 39.5 months on average to receive a diagnosis.

Researchers still have not found a way to tell us if and how fear of and negative attitudes toward dementia directly affect the daily lives of people with dementia. But a concept known as "identity threat," borrowed from more general studies of how stigma affects us, can be helpful here. Identity threat is just what it sounds like. It happens when someone's identity is threatened by stigma, either from the outside or from their own self-doubts that lead them to tumble toward a self-fulfilling prophecy. The damage can happen when the threat is greater than what the person's coping skills can handle. Things like being exposed to media images that reinforce stigmas (by, for example, watching a movie in which people with dementia are seen solely as objects of pity) or being compelled to reveal a stigmatized condition (by, for instance, being asked to take a cognitive test) can raise the identity threat level. When someone threatens our identity, our stress levels go up. For people with dementia, increases in stress can mean that valuable and already taxed cognitive resources get used up. People who are stigmatized are at greater risk for depression, hypertension, coronary heart disease, and stroke than people who aren't stigmatized.

How do we *learn* to stigmatize dementia? How do we *learn* negative attitudes toward aging and dementia? The same way we learn anything else—by watching and repeating. In still another study with Becca Levy on the team, researchers found that older adults who watched television had significantly worse attitudes about aging than those who did not. The good news is that Levy and colleagues also found that simply by *thinking critically* about what they were seeing, those same older adults could break television's spell. Those older viewers who kept a journal of their reactions to what they saw had less negative attitudes about aging and more negative attitudes about television itself. Some even vowed to stop watching it.

Encouraging media literacy about aging might well mitigate the health hazards of watching television. Encouraging people to turn off the television might just get a few more people out walking (and improving their physical and cognitive health) as well. But some care partners rely on the television to absorb the attention of their loved one with dementia, thereby allowing them critical moments of focus and rest during the day. Television can also be a vital source of news and information. Completely turning off the television might not be the right solution. I hold out hope that the images of aging and dementia in mass media can become more balanced. Much of this book is dedicated to

sharing complex stories of aging and dementia, stories that unfold in
senior center auditoriums as well as stadium-seating multiplexes. More
such stories are out there—and they need to find their way to more
people so that greater numbers of Americans learn what dementia is and
become aware that services and help are available and that a meaningful
life is possible with the right care and support systems.

> ABE: Why are you people avoiding me? Does my withered face remind you
> of the grim specter of Death?
>
> HOMER: (*pause*) Yes, but there's more. (*sits down on the couch*)
> Dad, I love you, but—(*angry*) you're a weird, sore-headed old crank
> and nobody likes you!
>
> ABE: Consarn it! I guess I am an old crank. But what am I going to do
> about it?
>
> (*On TV, mellow music plays and three old people drink Buzz Cola. Suddenly,
> they're transformed into partiers. An old man with an H. R. Beck guitar
> wears Hawaiian shorts.*)
>
> OLD MAN: One sip and I'm totally hip!
>
> ANNOUNCER: Buzz Cola. There's a little boogie in every bottle.
>
> ABE: Holy smokes, that's it! From now on I'm thinkin', actin', and lookin'
> young, and I'm gonna start with a bottle of Buzz Cola.
>
> (*grabs it from Homer, starts to chug*)
> Oh! Ah! Ow! The bubbles are burning my tongue! Ow! Oh! Water!
> Water!

Part Two

THE STORIES WE TELL ABOUT DEMENTIA IN POPULAR CULTURE

> ✎ The most erroneous stories are those we think we know best—and therefore never scrutinize or question.
>
> Steven Jay Gould

The stories we tell about dementia in the mainstream media create the backdrop against which we forge our understandings of and attitudes toward it. So what exactly *are* we seeing and hearing about memory loss in the mainstream media? Not much. In fact, there aren't many images of older people at all in popular culture. Estimates tell us that people over 65 are 17 percent of the population, yet they make up only 2 percent of characters on television. These 2 percent of characters are largely a blend of extremes; the absurdly fit, funny, and sexy or the severely disabled. Although the numbers of older characters will increase (and likely have since the 2 percent figure was derived) as marketers vie for the buying power of the growing numbers of people cresting 65, the way older people are depicted will likely remain the same, with the most extreme images appearing in commercials. The disparity in representation and the stereotyping on television are mirrored in popular film and mainstream magazines. One television studio executive rationalized the low percentage of elderly characters by explaining that young people don't want to watch older people, but older people remember being young and will watch younger people.

There is little information on the prevalence of imagery of dementia. Those numbers are hidden inside the figures of "negative" images and stereotypes of aging. But my interest isn't in the numbers. It doesn't take a hundred stories about dementia to create a paralyzing feeling of dread and to atrophy public will to change our broken system of long-term care; a few horrible images or the general absence of images can do the job just as effectively.

Dementia, particularly the most common form of dementia, Alzheimer's disease, began to appear on the public radar after the formation of the first national Alzheimer's association in 1980. The Alzheimer's Disease and Related Disorders Association (ADRDA), which changed its name to the Alzheimer's Association in 1988, took as one of its charges the challenge of raising public awareness of Alzheimer's disease. Their efforts bore early fruit in public service announcements with celebrities (like Jack Lemmon in 1982), Senate hearings, trade books, a pivotal "Dear Abby" column in 1980 (which generated more than 30,000 response letters), and mainstream magazine articles. These early efforts were meant to crack open a public space for the long, strange, almost unpronounceable word "Alzheimer's." If the association was to serve families (another goal), those families had to know the name of what they had and whom to call for help. If it was to raise money to find a cure (another goal), policy makers had to know it was a disease with dire individual, familial, and societal consequences.

Before the 1980s, as Jesse Ballenger adroitly shows in *Self, Senility, and Alzheimer's Disease in Modern America,* what we now know as dementia was largely thought of as "senility." In the scientific community, Alzheimer's disease was commonly thought of as a *disease* only if it hit someone in his or her 40s, 50s, or 60s, what is now considered the prime years of one's working and family life. To turn this ship around—to penetrate the American consciousness, to engage the country's political will, and to challenge scientific tradition—the message about Alzheimer's disease would have to be strong indeed.

And it was. "The Agony of Azheimer's Disease" reads the cover of *Newsweek* in 1984. The accompanying article is called "A Slow Death of the Mind." The Senate Subcommittee on Aging hearing in 1983 was called "Endless Night, Endless Mourning: Living with Alzheimer's." The tone of these early messages reverberates today. These stories figured dementia wholly as a tragedy, a tragedy for the persons with the disease, for families, and for society at large. They painted the disease with the largest brushes they could find, representing it as an epidemic with enormous financial costs that threaten the economic security of the country. Because the cost of care was imagined to be economically catastrophic, massive investment in a scientific solution was seen as the only real hope. Further, as Ballenger points out, the National Institute on Aging (NIA), founded in 1974, was deeply invested in these stories. NIA founders needed to separate normal "aging" from disease so that they might vie for research funds with other National Institutes of Health players. They picked Alzheimer's as their disease and were instrumental in shaping public messages about dementia during this time. In the 1980s, Alzheimer's as tragedy was the first and strongest story to emerge about it, and that story continues to dominate the headlines and movie and television screens today.

Dementia is associated with two types of tragic story. First, there is the one in which dementia is represented as a calamity that can only be eliminated if scientists are given enough time and money to find the cure. Second is the tale of the loss of an accomplished, inspiring person, a person slowly emptied out by a devastating illness. How do these stories work? And what experiences do they leave on the cutting room floor?

3

Memory Loss
in the Mainstream

Tightly Told Tragedies of Dementia
with Science as Hero

❧ *The Forgetting: A Portrait of Alzheimer's* is a 2-hour special aimed at helping people better understand and cope with the fearsome disease of
Alzheimer's. . . . The documentary is a dramatic, compassionate, all-
encompassing look at Alzheimer's that weaves together the history
and biology of the disease, the intense real-world experiences of
Alzheimer's patients and caregivers, and the race to find a cure.

The Forgetting

A prime example of dementia presented as tragedy is the 2004 documentary *The Forgetting*. The film, which premiered on PBS as a "common carriage" showing (scheduled by all stations across the country), is
based on David Shenk's book *The Forgetting: Alzheimer's, Portrait of an
Epidemic*, published in 2001. The book itself is full of nuance—it is
sober about the world of scientific inquiry into dementia; it puts Alzheimer's into a vivid, historical context; and it shares the hopes and feelings of people with dementia themselves. But the film sees Alzheimer's
in purely tragic terms—and depicts science as our one great hope to end
the pointless wasting of minds, lives, and money. Actress Linda Hunt
narrates the film, and her haunting voice sets the tone for the film.
Alzheimer's is a "slow and silent killer." It "draws the curtain over a patient's life and pulls family into its devastating grasp. . . . Fifteen years
ago, there were approximately 500,000 Americans with Alzheimer's.
Today there are 5 million." Produced and directed by Elizabeth Arledge,
The Forgetting played to eight million viewers and drew an estimated
one million people to the corresponding Web site in the first year. This
is far more than the estimated 100,000 copies of the book in circulation.

The film of *The Forgetting* tells the story of Alzheimer's disease by weaving together two tales: the scientific race to discover how the disease works and how to stop it, and the reason for that heartfelt race—the tremendous suffering of families and people with Alzheimer's. The metaphors for the disease are rather violent in the film. Dr. Rudolph Tanzi is an Alzheimer's researcher featured in the film and coauthor with Ann Parson of *Decoding Darkness,* a book chronicling the scientific quest for cure that was published in 2000. In the opening segment of the film, Tanzi's voice is heard over rapid, increasingly chaotic cuts of old family photos and home video. "Alzheimer's disease *robs* you of who you are," he says. "I don't think there's any greater fear for a person than to think I've lived my whole life accumulating all these memories, all of these value systems, all of this place and my family and a society. And here's a disease that is just going to come in and every single day just *rip* out the connections, just *tear* out the seams[,] that actually define who I am as a person" (the italics are mine).

David Shenk is also interviewed in this opening sequence. Invoking imagery of a nuclear holocaust, he describes Alzheimer's disease: "[It] has just mushroomed in just the last 15 years from this relatively rare disorder into this extremely common phenomenon. . . . We're in the middle of an epidemic. We absolutely have to stop this disease. There's just no choice. As a nation, as an economy, as a civilization, we have to end it now." The film's language and use of numbers can be a little misleading. "Epidemic" has multiple meanings. It can mean "contagious." It can also mean "excessively prevalent." Certainly Shenk means the latter, but the panic associated with the first meaning lends weight to his description (and the subtitle of his book: *Portrait of an Epidemic*). Further, the claim that 15 years ago there were only 500,000 cases and now there are 5 million doesn't take into account the fact that 15 years ago, Alzheimer's disease was largely considered "senility" or senile dementia and was not widely diagnosed. Most researchers agree that this dramatic boost in the numbers is due to a combination of more people living longer and a greater willingness among doctors to diagnose the condition.

The Forgetting's story of the scientific race for answers is riveting. The film follows Dr. Steven DeKosky, then at the University of Pittsburgh, from his visits with patients, to his lab, and through his quest to find a substance that helps researchers see the impact of the disease on the brain via neuroimaging. The stakes are clearly high—families are suffering greatly. And when DeKosky tells how their long-shot efforts paid off, you want to "high-five" his entire scientific team. There are multiple approaches to the science of Alzheimer's (Is it the plaques? Is it the tangles? Is it a gene?), and the reputation and financial futures of labs and scientists are at stake. But in the film version of *The Forgetting*, these affable scientists are clearly caring people, and they put aside their personal interests to collaborate on the quest to find a cure.

To tell a story that centers on the hope of scientific research and the urgency of supporting such research, Arledge presents the experience of Alzheimer's in a particular way. All of the people with Alzheimer's whom we meet in the film are deep into the disease process. There are no flashes of lucidity or grace here. Arledge creates a sharp contrast between the person as he or she is now and the person he or she was (which is conveyed through family stories, videos, and photographs). The film introduces us to three women: an adventurous, young woman fond of dancing; a beloved and capable mother; and a relatively young woman (40s) who shares her freshly discovered genetic fate with a local news station. These strong, lively women are now lost to the "darkness" of the disease. Daughters quietly pray for their mother to be relieved of her suffering. A husband acknowledges that a cure won't help his wife now and tells of his grandson's confusion over his grandmother's erratic bursts of anger. Siblings of the now 54-year-old woman deep in Alzheimer's agonize over the fact that at any moment one of them could be next. And by show's end, one of them is.

Arledge's message in *The Forgetting* is clear. The dramatic cut from family despair to the inspiring, scientific search for cure makes it evident that in her view the most important thing we can do is push for a scientific cure. It is this kind of message that gets people to write a senator in support of increasing federal research dollars to find a cure. Two articles from the broadly circulated news magazines *Time* and *Newsweek* in 2000 adopted a similar storyline. The *Newsweek* article, published in January, begins with a paragraph that traps readers in the experience of Alzheimer's by addressing them in the rare second-person voice, describing the early suspicions that "something might be wrong" and how "pretty soon . . . you're painfully aware" of what will become a "silent stupor" complete with "bedsores and diaper rash." "Death, when it comes," the paragraph closes, "is a formality." It is a gut-wrenching introduction to the disease, which it depicts as a common, meaningless, quick, and horrifying journey. The horror of the disease, as rendered through a made-up scenario, is countered by the impending and exciting high-stakes race for cure: "The longer we live, the more likely we are to contract this devastating disease. But recent discoveries are bringing scientists closer than ever to a cure."

Like Arledge's film version of *The Forgetting*, the *Newsweek* article tells the story of disease's journey from relative obscurity ("Alzheimer's was rare when scientists first identified it a century ago") to household name ("The United States case load is expected to explode"). The article makes no mention of the fact that the original diagnosis applied only to people who were under 60, still only a slim percentage of the number of Alzheimer's cases today. The other story of Alzheimer's science, published in *Time* in July, invokes the same metaphors as the *Newsweek* piece. The number of cases in this "epidemic" will "explode." The scientific war between the "Baptists" and the "Tauists" (those banking on beta amyloid plaques as the cause versus those who insist Alzheimer's is caused by the tau-related tangles) is depicted as moving us toward a cure "sooner than one might have dared hope."

The metaphor of "darkness" is common in these stories of scientific discovery; thus, for example, Tanzi and Parson's title, *Decoding Darkness*. This image of "darkness" is a particularly powerful motif for the scientific story because it works so well against the visuals provided by the brain imaging techniques that start to become common around this time. "Imagine your brain is a house filled with lights," the *Time* article opens. "Now imagine someone turning off the lights one by one . . . and you succumb to the spreading darkness." The *Newsweek* article features a brain scan image that shows little color and appears "dark." It is captioned "The dying of the light." *The Forgetting* closes with Linda Hunt's voice commenting on the birthday party of the newly diagnosed brother from the family haunted by the early-onset form of Alzheimer's. "By his next birthday, Butch might not recognize everyone he loves. And like millions of other families, [they] will watch as his mind fades into the darkness of forgetting."

The majority of mainstream media stories about Alzheimer's disease, particularly in magazines and newspapers, cluster around scientific breakthroughs, likely due to the bench depth of public relations personnel at pharmaceutical companies and the growing strength of the national Alzheimer's Association. One study of popular magazines found that just a handful of articles appeared in the 1990s. In 2000 and 2001, however, 17 articles appeared, which was the same period during which the FDA approved the drug Exelon and just a few years after Aricept was approved to treat mild to moderate Alzheimer's disease (1996). The 25 articles that appeared between 1991 and 2001 were told almost exclusively from the medical perspective. The disease was described as "fearsome, relentless, and aggressive." Not one article featured the perspective of the person experiencing the disease.

This was a time of battle cry, of ringing the alarm about Alzheimer's disease as loudly as possible. As I've said before, the experience of dementia is hard. It can take a heavy emotional, physical, and financial toll on families. Certainly, getting the word out about the disease is crucial if our goal is to raise funds to study it and to encourage people to find their way get to help. But it's important that we see what gets left on the cutting room floor during the making of such tragic stories. And it's important to acknowledge that the tragic story, in which science is the white knight, tells only part of it.

There is another kind of tragic story, one that doesn't focus on science for hope. How do these stories work? How do they differ from those situated within a medical framework?

4

Tightly Told Tragedies of Dementia

Then versus Now

> [Alzheimer's] robs not only the person who has it but the family members—their memories of who that person was are threatened to be replaced by the stranger that comes to live in that body.
>
> Leeza Gibbons

The story of dementia as tragedy also appears in books, television shows, and movies that aren't focused on the scientific promise for cure. In this group of stories, like in the film version of *The Forgetting*, there is a sharp contrast between who the person *was then,* and who the person *is now.* These stories climax in a moment when the two worlds (then and now) come together to reach some sort of harmony. This climax is commonly a moment of sudden lucidity—in which a woman suddenly recognizes her husband, or a father clearly expresses himself to his son—but can also be a moment of clarity for the caregiver about his or her perspective on the disease.

As in Greek and Shakespearian tragedy, in which a fall is more pronounced when taken from the height of kings, these stories most commonly involve people who stand out, people with extraordinary hearts and minds. "Alzheimer's has hit Hollywood in the heart" was the pitch of the commercial break of the Maury Povich show in 1992, which featured actresses Shelly Fabares and Angie Dickinson. "They never thought it could happen to them," said Povich, suggesting that celebrities, our modern-day kings and queens, thought their status would keep them arm's length from dementia. Instead, it hit Fabares's mother and Dickinson's sister.

On a 1987 episode of *Oprah,* a husband and his children shared their story of losing his wife and their mother on a trip to New York City. It's terrible to imagine the elegant Mr. Gilbert, methodically walking the streets, taping up posters, looking for his wife, replaying the words of police that the longer it takes, the less likely it is she'll be found alive. A random stroke of luck (and the help of a homeless woman) led him to his wife, who was resting in a park, miles from where she'd last been seen. Mr. Gilbert was careful to establish that his wife was very intelligent, that she worked at the Library of Congress. His emotions were raw, and as a viewer, I thought he was simply pointing out that he never expected this to happen to her, to him, to his family. Certainly dementia is no easier when it strikes someone less conventionally "smart"—someone, say, with developmental disabilities or with Down syndrome, for example. But stories of everyday folks with everyday lives and intelligence aren't as dramatic and their prime-time appeal isn't as high, so we seldom see them.

Perhaps the most dramatic mainstream story of this kind—emphasizing a Shakespearian fall from great heights—came in 1994, when the Reagan family shared the news that former President Ronald Reagan had been diagnosed with Alzheimer's disease. This story barely needed explanation. It was enough to say "President Reagan" and "Alzheimer's" in the same sentence to convey the magnitude of his tragic fall. The news coverage—national, local, urban, rural—did more to bring the term "Alzheimer's" into the consciousness of Americans than any movie, magazine article, public service announcement, or book. The major news coverage burst forth again in 2004, when Reagan died and the Alzheimer's Association was designated as one of the three official memorial charities.

One of the first mainstream films about Alzheimer's follows a high-stakes then/now tragic storyline. Starring Joann Woodward, *Do You Remember Love?* appeared on television in 1987. Bright piano music opens the film behind images of Barbara (Woodward) and George Hollis (Richard Kiley) out for a vigorous, uphill bike ride through lush, late summer foliage. The opening collage of images establishes their lives as filled with fun (they joke about fishing), romance (complete with fireside sexual innuendo: "I'll keep you warm"), and intellectual challenge (they recite poems to each other over wine). The first sign of difficulty comes early in the film, when a friend points out that Barbara, a professor of poetry, is headed the wrong way to her classroom. In the next scene, we learn that Barbara is exceptional—she's up for tenure (without a PhD!) and is being considered for a prestigious Longfellow Award for poetry. Right away, we know these two themes—her increasing confusion and her increasing professional recognition—are headed for collision.

And in the final moments of *Do You Remember Love?* they do. Having lost her job, been taken into custody for making a spectacle of herself in a public park, and alienated her closest friends, Barbara wins the Longfellow Award. Her family rallies around her, sitting in support while she goes up to accept the award on her own. When she fumbles, her husband joins her onstage, explaining his wife's challenges to the audience without a trace of shame. Written and produced before science had made much progress on Alzheimer's, *Do You Remember Love?* is the tragic story of a bright, poetic light burning out before its time and her family's journey toward acceptance. It edges toward melodrama in its predictably drawn characters (there's a good professor and a bad professor), but it was also enormously brave—it tackled an illness almost unheard of at the time and included a scene in the couple's bed in which Woodward screams at her husband, "Give it to me!" The blend of raw anger, sexual desire, illness, and older actors should have been enough to make most networks pull the plug.

John Bayley's memoir *Elegy for Iris* and Nicholas Sparks's novel *The Notebook,* both published in 1999, share similar storylines. Bayley's book tells of a woman elevated by a great mind (Iris Murdoch) and Sparks's of a woman, Allie, filled with a great love (for *The Notebook*'s fictional husband, Noah). Both books were also made into major motion pictures. *Iris* premiered in 2001 (the year the book version of *The Forgetting* was published), and *The Notebook* premiered in 2004 (the year *The Forgetting* appeared on PBS).

Iris juxtaposes the philosophical language and deep thought of the young Iris as she navigates her world of classrooms, dinner parties, and gatherings of great minds with the older Iris, enrapt by the Teletubbies and reading for a doctor as her words drop "like dead birds." The film is beautifully made and acted (by Kate Winslet, Judi Dench, and Jim Broadbent, among others). It tells the story of Murdoch's life and recounts Bayley's struggle to find reason or meaning—some sort of sense—in the dissonance between her life before and her life with Alzheimer's. John Bayley's character in the book and in the film ultimately concludes that Iris was always a mystery in his life. She would disappear for periods of time, had affairs with figures (men and women) who remained shadowy to him. Murdoch's Alzheimer's seems to perpetuate that mystery. Except rather than hiding behind closed doors, Iris hid deep in the recesses of her mind. The story of *Iris* is one of tremendous loss, not just for the person of Iris Murdoch but also for humankind—who lost what she might have created had she not developed Alzheimer's. For John Bayley, however, the book and the film tell the story of a growing clarity. As Iris moved deeper into Alzheimer's and her world narrowed, her need for him and his role in her life finally became clear to him. This free spirit and great mind finally needed his care.

Science provides little help for Iris, and neither the book nor the film expresses hope. The doctors have no medicines to offer, and their only advice is a cold slap of reality—"and it *will* get worse." The book and film are particularly sobering in light of the latest scientific messages—that cognitive exercise and social networks can help build "cognitive reserves" to stave off the effects of dementia. One can't imagine someone more cognitively fit or socially supported than Iris Murdoch.

I had a love/hate relationship with the film *The Notebook*. I vividly remember standing in the line for tickets for a Tuesday afternoon matinee. The teenage girls at the front of line asked for tickets to *The Notebook*. The people behind them, who looked to be a 60-year-old man and his 80-year-old mother, asked for tickets to the same film. I got my tickets and made my way down the winding corridors to the theater. There were maybe 20 people there. Half were high schoolers, drawn to the film to see Ryan Gosling and Rachel McAdams, two young rising stars. The other half were over 60, drawn to the film, I imagine, to watch James Garner and Gena Rowlands play the older counterparts to Gosling and McAdams, whose love perseveres through class differences, family pressures, and what the film calls "senile dementia."

And then there was me. I went to *The Notebook* to see how it portrayed the experience of dementia. What story was it telling? I loved the fact that there were equal numbers of people under 20 and over 60 crunching overpriced popcorn at the same afternoon matinee. Such common meeting grounds are rare. But with what story would the audience walk away?

In *The Notebook,* a dapper, elderly gentleman (James Garner) reads to a well-coifed but somewhat blank-looking woman (Gena Rowlands) in a stunning, white plantation-like nursing home. The story he tells her chronicles a passionate love affair between a young couple, Noah and Allie, who must cross the tracks several times to find each other. As the film shifts between the young lovers and the older couple, we gradually realize that the older Noah is reading the story of their lives to Allie in the hopes that the strength of their passion will bring her out of the fog of dementia. Noah's story seems to entertain Allie, but her eyes show she has no memory of her husband—then or now.

The Notebook stretches our understanding of dementia to the limit. The older Allie is gorgeous (at least 2 hours of primping per day would be my guess), and she follows the story Noah reads to her quite easily. She asks coherent questions. She doesn't stumble over words. She simply can't remember him. The film suggests that the strength of her husband's love is enough to pull her out of her confusion for several brief moments and one rather extended moment. At film's end, the strength of the love they share is enough to pull them both, simultaneously it seems, into a peaceful sleep from which they never awaken. This heavily sentimentalized film was hard for me to watch. But at least it was democratic. We view the young couple's story through the same rose-tinted lens as that of the old couple. The hope here was not in a cure but rather that a tremendously powerful love could bring about one last moment of clarity and then pull one into death and relieve one's suffering.

The storylines of these three films (*The Notebook, Iris,* and *Do You Remember Love?*) are similar. They tell a tragic tale of loss, a fall from heights of greatness (intellect, talent, and/or love). The husband faces the challenge of helping his wife through this loss. Will he be able to handle it? Will he protect or even "rescue" her, as James Garner does? None of the husbands is a saint. John Bayley's housekeeping habits are downright disgusting. But each finds nobility in the final moments of these loss stories. The assumption is that these great minds and great loves have been violated. And we have been violated alongside them. They've lost their dignity, and we've lost the creative contributions they could have made if they had aged into a natural death in late life without dementia. Let me note here that I admire some of these films and that I agree that the experience of dementia can be tragic, for many reasons. My goal in looking closely at the narrative structure of these stories is to discover what is left out of the stories. Is the experience of dementia *only* a tragedy?

The tragedy narrative has a visual counterpart in advertising. In the national Alzheimer's Association's highly visible "Warning Signs" campaign from 1993, a graying woman who appears to be in her late 60s looks downward at nothing in particular. She is alone. She stands next to a mirror, but her reflection is deliberately blurred—the washes of light and dark just barely suggest a human image. The ad's story is that Alzheimer's is a lonely, alienating experience in which the body is present but the ability to "reflect" is gone.

Another series of ads for the Alzheimer's Association emphasizes the tragedy of forgetting pivotal moments in our lives. "Imagine not re-membering your own daughter's name. For thousands of women each year, it's becoming a reality." The text is accompanied by an image of a young, beaming bride standing next to her mother. "Who doesn't re-member the sight of that 3-year-old boy saluting his father's casket as it passed? At last count, about 4 million people," reads the text of another ad that is accompanied by an image of a young John Kennedy at the bottom of the page in a spotlight that looks like it is disappearing before our eyes. In these ads, forgetting is itself a tragedy.

In contrast, another series of ads from the Alzheimer's Association in 2005 tells a different story. An image of a mother and two grown daugh-ters playing with a dog is captioned "Alzheimer's doesn't mean you for-get how to care." Here, it is clear that memory loss is complicated and that some kinds of memory, and one's sense of self, remain. Other cap-tions in this series include "Alzheimer's doesn't mean you forget how to hug," with a photograph of an older couple relishing a warm embrace, and "Alzheimer's doesn't mean you forget how to play," with a photo-graph of an African American grandfather, father, and son on a boat, laughing and fishing. This ad campaign tells a different story about mem-ory loss; one that suggests that tragedy might not capture the *whole* story of dementia. After 2003, more complex stories of memory loss and de-mentia begin to appear in mainstream media. Some of them feature older people—some of them, surprisingly, feature fish.

5

Not So Tightly Tragic
Stories That Imagine Something More

✌ I think all we can aspire to in this situation is a little bit of grace.

Away from Her

The experience of dementia entails significant losses. There can be fear, anxiety, confusion, personality change, and sometimes hallucinations. It is the stories of these many losses that we hear most often. But is there *more* than loss in dementia? Are there experiences in dementia that don't fit into the tightly told tragedies? In my conversations with Roger and Rocille, I am struck by their determination to remain deeply engaged with life. They attend meetings, services, classes, parties. They traveled to Sicily. "Roger and I have not changed our philosophy of life," said Rocille. "We're still going on." There are pop culture stories and images that capture the everyday moments that can be deeply meaningful and that focus on the possibility of growth in the midst of an experience riddled with loss. These stories suggest that one's sense of "self" is greater than the sum of one's memories.

David Shenk's book *The Forgetting: Alzheimer's, Portrait of an Epidemic* (2001) deftly weaves a story of scientific discovery and anguish with mankind's epic quest for meaning in the face of loss. Shenk shares eloquent observations of people with dementia as well as those of caregivers, scientists, and some of Western culture's great philosophers and literary minds. In doing so, he sets what we now understand to be Alzheimer's disease in the well-laid tracks of Plato, Plutarch, St. Augustine, William Shakespeare, Jonathan Swift, Mark Twain, Henry David Thoreau, Ralph Waldo Emerson, Friedrich Nietzsche, Frederick Olmsted, and Viktor Frankl. The result is comforting. Shenk shows us that this awkward-sounding disease, first "diagnosed" in 1906, isn't new at all. And over several continents and several thousand years, it has inspired some of the deepest thinking about the meaning of human existence.

Shenk closes *The Forgetting* with the image of Morris Freidell, a former professor of sociology, searching for ways to live and grow in the face of his dementia diagnosis. Shenk paints an image of Freidell standing in a sea of poster presentations at a national scientific conference on dementia—a lonely voice for those living with the disease. Could the scientific story (of tragedy, objectivity, and abstract molecules) and the human story (of striving for meaning and purpose) coexist? Shenk writes: "I still respected that dichotomy, still feared the disease, and still hoped for a cure, of course—as did Morris. But I also now realized that the story of Alzheimer's is in some ways exactly the opposite of my original premise: It is a condition specific to humans and as old as humanity that, like nothing else, acquaints us with life's richness by ever so gradually drawing down the curtains. Only through modern science has this poignancy been reduced to a plain horror, an utterly unhuman circumstance."

The film, as we have seen, tells a purely dark tale. How could the book and the film tell such different stories? Part of it has to do with the medium. Both the book and the film recount the high-stakes scientific gambles on the road to finding a cure. But a book has the luxury of length, something that enabled Shenk to include more nuance about the daily lives of families dealing with Alzheimer's. Naomi Boak, the executive producer of *The Forgetting,* readily acknowledges that the purpose of a 90-minute film is to leave a strong impression. "Films can't be that complex," said Boak. "It's not how we process information. We try to leave an impression with the film and then have more detailed information in the website or book." The Web site (www.pbs.org/theforgetting) tells a story of Alzheimer's and memory loss much more akin to the book by including stories by people with dementia alongside those of great thinkers, scientists, and caregivers.

But other films do manage to make a strong impression *and* focus less on the tragic side. The 2006 film *Away from Her* shares Shenk's desire to see something more in dementia. Based on the powerful short story "The Bear Came over the Mountain," by Alice Munro, *Away from Her* tells the story of the relationship between Fiona (Julie Christie) and Grant (Gordon Pinsent), a couple who appear to be in their late 60s or early 70s. The film opens with Fiona casually putting a frying pan in the freezer. When she leaves the room, Grant silently removes the pan and puts it away. And so it begins.

"I think all we can aspire to in this situation is a little bit of grace," Fiona whispers to Grant, calming his frantic desire to fight the disease.

This phrase captures a significant shift in mainstream stories about dementia. Rather than focus on tragic decline, *Away from Her* looks for moments of grace, eschewing the linear plot line that seeks climax and resolution. "Grace" has a variety of meanings—depending on your religious framework (or lack thereof). In one sense of the word, to have grace is to be sanctified by God. In turn, "sanctified" means to be "set apart to a sacred purpose or religious use." If dementia (or other earthly conditions) discourages you from believing in God, this definition can still be useful—moments of "grace" might also be seen as those that provide a sense of purpose or that can be of use to one's self and other people.

Away from Her has its share of loss. Fiona loses her conscious memory of her family history. "They've kept it just as it was," she says of her grandmother's cabin, in which you can feel the presence of multiple generations in the old woodwork. She has forgotten that she has lived there for the past 20 years. Fiona also seems to forget her life with her husband, whom she mistakes for a new resident at the nursing home—trying to comfort him, she says, "You'll get used to it." Grant loses the intimacy he and Fiona shared. Other than occasionally cutting to hazy, romantic images of Fiona as a young woman (made to look like old home movies), the film doesn't spend much time on Fiona as she was "then." It's not clear if she worked at all, and her family stories are not even broadly sketched.

Instead, director Sarah Polley focuses on the *now*, which is like an alien planet on which we must learn not to look into the future for anything—narrative meaning, progress, or hope. Instead, in this world in which the present and past overwrite each other, we find grace in beauty, wonder, kindness, and raw human connection. On a walk with Grant, Fiona bends down to look at a bright flower and laughs. "When I turn away, I forget yellow. Yellow is new every time. There's something delicious in oblivion," she marvels. And later, having become lost in the snowy woods, Fiona collapses. Facing the sky, she relaxes and appears on the verge of making a snow angel. Her expression is a complex swirl of both fear (How will I get home? What is happening to me?) and acceptance (Look at the beauty around me). Grant reveals a similar complexity. Rather than succumb to his jealousies, Grant encourages the intimacy between Fiona and another resident named Aubrey, because it clearly comforts her. Grant himself finds a frenetic comfort in a sexual relationship with Aubrey's wife.

I was surprised that the film, which takes such pains to avoid traditional plot lines in the dementia story, ends with a moment of lucidity. Grant, who has fought to return Aubrey to the nursing home in the hope that that might bring Fiona out of her depression, is shocked to find that Fiona suddenly recognizes Grant as her husband. As Aubrey sits outside the door of their room, the couple suddenly seems back to "normal." But this is just another moment of grace; a gift perhaps to Grant but not a return to their relationship. The screen fades to black rather than resolve the moment.

Away from Her caught fire in the press. Prominent articles and reviews appeared in every major newspaper and extensive television and radio interviews were conducted with the film's director, Sarah Polley, and the film's well-known stars like Olympia Dukakis. The story of the film in the press revolves largely around the fact that Polley, still in her 20s when she made it, chose the subject matter of Alzheimer's for her directorial debut. "What could possibly have interested such a young, talented woman in *that?*" is the subtext of the press coverage. Polley's response is that she read the short story just after she'd gotten married. The early days of a relationship, when both partners are woozy with passion, didn't seem nearly as rich to her as the later days, when a lifetime of hopes, hurts, dreams, regrets, and habits play themselves out. Alzheimer's is more a complicating factor in the story of Fiona and Grant's lifelong relationship than a story in and of itself.

There is something *more* to the story of *Away from Her* than dementia. One critic described the film as "less a drama about Alzheimer's disease than a cinematic poem of love and loss." *Away from Her* is also a story about how young people *should* take interest in the lives of the old.

6

Not Tragic at All

Stories about Memory Loss without the Old

🪰 HENRY: And now, I would like to introduce to you our most distin-
guished clinical subject . . . Tom.

TOM: Hi. I'm Tom. Cool flip-flops. Where'd you get them?

HENRY: You like those? It's interesting. I was on the North Shore—

TOM: Hi, I'm Tom.

HENRY: Hi.

DOCTOR: Tom lost part of his brain . . . in a hunting accident. His
memory lasts 10 seconds.

TOM: I was in an accident? That's terrible.

DOCTOR: Don't worry. You'll get over it in seconds.

TOM: Get over it? I mean, what happened? Did I get shot in the
brain—? Hi, I'm Tom.

50 First Dates

There are stories that focus on the tragic components of dementia and
memory loss. There are stories, like *Away from Her,* that look for something *more* than tragedy in memory loss. Then there are those stories
that look for something more than tragedy in memory loss—but forget
something crucial: older people.

We've all seen them. Gilligan gets hit on the head with a coconut.
Any number of soap opera stars wake up after some sort of accident to
find they have no idea who they are or with whom they've had sex. The
trope of amnesia is common in any era. It enables writers (good and
bad) to ask the age-old question, "Who am I?" (or "Who is my family?"
or "Who is my community?") in a plot line in which the audience and
the main character are on a parallel path of discovery. Neither the audience nor the main character knows the answer. Amnesia also serves a
classic American plot line—leaving behind the past (the old country
and the old self) and remaking one's self in a new land. Susan Sontag

puts it another way, describing America as "an evangelical church prone to announcing radical endings and brand-new beginnings." But the overwhelming numbers of mainstream films in the last 20 years predicated on memory loss is enough to make you think Americans should wear helmets 24/7. What's behind this wave of amnesia films? Are the stories about young people with memory loss different from those about older people? If so, why?

There have been two significant waves of memory loss imagery in U.S. culture in the last 65 years. Around the time of World War II, a cluster of films were produced in which the trope of memory loss was associated with imagining how we might "forget" the brutal memories of war and move on, as individuals and as a country. War-era films with this theme include *Random Harvest* (1942), *Spellbound* (1945), *Blue Dahlia* (1946), *Deadline at Dawn* (1946), *Somewhere in the Night* (1946), and *The Great Dictator* (1940). The memory loss in these films typically stemmed from a rough knock on the head, an emotional trauma, or possibly both.

The more recent wave of memory loss imagery has its roots in the 1980s but hit full force beginning in the mid-1990s. These films range across numerous genres, from comedy (*50 First Dates* [2004]) to indy/cult (*Desperately Seeking Susan* [1985]; *Memento* [2000]; *Eternal Sunshine of the Spotless Mind* [2004]; *Mulholland Drive* [2001]; *Nurse Betty* [2000]) and from action (*The Long Kiss Goodnight* [1996]; *The Bourne Identity* [2002]; *The Bourne Supremacy* [2004]; *The Bourne Ultimatum* [2007]) to science fiction/fantasy (*Total Recall* [1990]; *The Matrix* [1999]; *Vanilla Sky* [2001]; *Paycheck* [2003]) to drama/romance (*The Majestic* [2001]; *A Very Long Engagement* [2004]).

What is triggering this current fascination with memory loss? Writers who take notice of the phenomenon, like John Leland (*New York Times* [2001]), Lev Grossman (*Time* [2004]), Andy Seiler (*USA Today* [2002]), and Terrence Rafferty (*New York Times* [2003]), credit a wide variety of cultural influences. Leland points to the dizzy economic excesses of the 1990s: "Dot-com diehards crowed that the business cycle no longer existed, and the exuberance of the market allowed anyone to believe the past was irrelevant." Leland also suggests that new technologies are making us anxious about our identity, describing how "identity became fluid, as anyone who has ever gone into a chat room knows. Memory could be erased with the stroke of a computer key." Similarly, Grossman asks, "If our minds are rippable, mixable and burnable as an

MP3, how can we ever be sure we know who we are? There's something profoundly sinister and infectious about the idea, and it's a virus we caught from our computers." Leland sums it up well: "In a culture obsessed with individuality, what could be more horrifying than to lose one's identity?" Rafferty also credits our tendency as a country to ignore the past in our obsession with instant gratification: "It's at least arguable that the movies' current fascination with amnesia reflects a growing sentiment that living ahistorically is not all it's been cracked up to be—that our past, as [Philip K.] Dick warned, has been hijacked, and we want it back. After the long, rough night that this new millennium has so far been, maybe we're all desperately trying to remember who we are."

I agree with their observations. But there is also an elephant in the room that none of these astute cultural critics even mentions in passing: the dramatic increase in both the number of people diagnosed with Alzheimer's disease and our awareness of the disease since the 1980s. Nor do these critics point to the aging of the baby boomers and their potential connection to memory loss. Many producers, directors, and writers are likely dealing with aging parents. Some of them are no doubt, consciously or subconsciously, questioning the state of their own cognitive abilities. The films, which do not treat the theme of memory loss as an age-related issue, might be avoiding direct representation of a phenomenon that frightens so many people so much.

In the contemporary wave of memory loss films, as in their World War II–era counterparts, memory loss is most commonly caused by physical or emotional trauma. Second most common are science fiction–oriented films, which tend toward scenarios in which memory loss is forced on characters by technological innovation or oppressive regimes (*The Matrix* series, *Total Recall*, etc.). In *Eternal Sunshine of the Spotless Mind*, for example, characters "elect" to undergo memory loss by having an ethically nebulous outpatient surgical procedure performed on them.

Sci-fi images aside, how common is amnesia? Memory loss associated with a bump on the head or psychological trauma, the most common type of memory loss depicted in this recent wave, can be "anterograde" (forgetting what takes place *after* the injury) and "retrograde" (forgetting what took place *before* the injury). It is debatable whether retrograde amnesia exists. Anterograde amnesia related to head trauma is uncommon, possibly limited to several hundred cases per year in the United States. Transient global amnesia is the temporary loss of all memory. It is extremely rare in the case of head injury and usually clears up in several hours. "Most of what I see in the movies on amnesia is preposterous," said David A. Hovda, director of the UCLA Brain Injury Research Center. "The odds of a really widespread memory loss from injury are minuscule. From an injury that leaves the person otherwise all right, that's pretty much unheard of."

Although amnesia is rare in everyday life, it is rampant in pop culture imagery. Dementia, on the other hand, which affects some 5 million people in the United States alone, is a major theme in only three mainstream films. As opposed to amnesia, Alzheimer's is neither sudden nor uniform, making it distinctly lacking in "cinematic flair." Of course, dementia also most commonly affects older adults, whom the entertainment industry tends to view as the third rail of blockbuster appeal. And while young people with amnesia can suddenly "wake up" for a happy ending, those in late life have limited time to undergo the potential positive transformation that a clean start can bring.

In the recent wave of mainstream films, amnesia operates on the level of cultural metaphor. But what does it stand for? There is a group of films that worry over our ability to manipulate human memory through technology. There are films that see memory loss as a positive opportunity for a fresh start in life and for living fully in the present— Sontag's "brand-new beginnings." There are films that look for the purpose of a life without memory and others that see memory loss as comic and frustrating but ultimately not debilitating. And of course, some films mix their metaphors.

What are the films? *The Bourne Identity* (2002), *The Bourne Supremacy* (2004), and *The Bourne Ultimatum* (2007) are action films in which Jason Bourne (Matt Damon) is a government-trained assassin who, thanks to a traumatic blow to the head (possibly several), has a chance to untangle the ethical snarls of his job by doing the right thing as he simultaneously uncovers his old identity and builds a new one.

The Majestic is a drama in which a car accident gives Peter Appleton (Jim Carrey), a B-movie writer of questionable character, the chance to start life over after he forgets his identity and is warmly taken in as a small town's long-lost son and war hero. After his memory returns, he struggles with his guilty secret and his desire to keep his new identity. Eventually, he comes clean, gets the girl, and regains the trust of the town, integrating his old and new lives in the process.

50 First Dates is a romantic comedy in which a car accident renders a young woman named Lucy (Drew Barrymore) unable to process short-term memory (anterograde amnesia). She lives in a 24-hour cycle before her memories of the day are wiped clean as she sleeps, beginning her own *Groundhog Day* the next morning. With the help of the clever and love-struck Henry Roth (Adam Sandler), Lucy discovers the joy of living in the present.

Compare these films with those that present memory loss as a tragedy, like *Iris* and *The Notebook*. In these films, the main character begins as a whole person, the product of a lifetime of experiences and accomplishments, and slowly unravels, sometimes taking those who care for him or her along for the downward ride. Without the promise of "new beginnings," this plot line is the antithesis of the classic American narrative.

One popular mainstream film creates its own genre. It is a tragedy in which the main character loses himself when he loses his memory. But he finds a unique way to link his past, present, and future—revenge and murder. Whenever I tell people that I write about images of memory loss, they ask: "Have you seen *Memento?* Isn't it great? I loved it!" I don't understand why people love this movie. It's not that I'm a snob; I loved the *Bourne* trilogy. It's not that I'm too serious; I truly enjoyed *50 First Dates*. *Memento* is the story of Leonard Shelby (Guy Pearce), a man who loses his memory after a blow to the head during a robbery attempt in which his wife is raped and killed. He vows revenge but has no memory of anything after the crime (anterograde amnesia). How can one solve a crime and exact revenge without memory? How can he trust his memory of the crime itself? Might *he* have done it? Did he imagine it? Did his wife just *leave* him? The movie is cleverly crafted. It begins at the end of the story and moves backward until the opening scene of the film—which was so confusing to the audience and Shelby alike—makes sense. The plot structure brings the audience into the experience of memory loss.

Each scene of *Memento* starts with Shelby waking up. When he looks around the room, neither he nor the audience knows how he got there, where he is, or what day it is. Shelby tattoos key facts and feelings on his body—in a sort of extreme post-it note reminder system. At a certain point in the course of the film, we realize Shelby has *already* killed the man responsible for his wife's death. And then Shelby and the viewers realize something else. Living without memory is bearable only if one has a strong sense of purpose. Shelby deliberately manipulates the facts (his tattoos) to point to another perpetrator. By planting hints suggesting that another person was responsible for his wife's death, Shelby keeps his purpose—to exact revenge. And he kills again. Essentially, *Memento* tells us that living a life without functional memory is worse than being a serial killer.

Finally, one mainstream film sees memory loss not as neither tragedy nor as a celebration of new beginnings (for young people) but as a disability that brings some benefits along with some plot complications. Again, however, the character with memory loss is not an older adult. It's not even human. It is an animated blue fish named Dory.

In Pixar's *Finding Nemo* (2003), Dory describes her ailment as "short-term memory loss," which is something that she thinks runs in her family. But she can't quite remember if that's true. Dory's positive attitude and lack of inhibitions (it seems that she forgets to be afraid) make her the better half of a team whose mission is to find Nemo. Dory's short-term memory loss is a complicating factor, one of many obstacles to the completion of the film's classic hero's journey plot line. But it does not threaten her sense of self or stop the forward progression of the plot. Instead, *Finding Nemo* casts memory loss as a disability to be managed.

Dory is blue, with no visible signs of gender or age, other than those suggested by her association with the actress who plays her "voice," Ellen DeGeneres. In fact, the only visible references to age in the film come in the form of offspring, who are small and somewhat pudgy compared to their parents, and the well-known actors we see in our mind's eye who play the parents and other adult fish, including Albert Brooks (Nemo's father, Marlin), Willem Dafoe (Gil), and Allison Janney (Peach), to mention a few. Even Crush, a sea turtle said to be 150 years old, bears no telltale, anthropomorphized markings of age such as a slow gait, a wobbly voice, or outdated speech or appearance (in contrast to the stooped and wrinkled aging ants in *A Bug's Life,* another Pixar film). Marlin, Nemo's father, is haunted by his memory of the loss of his wife and all but one of what appeared to be hundreds of eggs ("kids") to a barracuda. The experience makes Marlin a hypercautious parent, filled with fear that another mishap will destroy what remains of his two-fish family. Because Dory has no memory of fear, she makes the perfect comic foil to Marlin. While Dory's constant repetition drives Marlin crazy, her lack of inhibitions and her trusting nature enable them to progress in their quest. They are a team. They rescue each other. They push each other along on their journey until they witness what they believe is the death of Nemo. His hopes squelched, Marlin thanks Dory and heads home.

> MARLIN: Dory, if it wasn't for you, I never even would have made it here. So thank you.
>
> DORY: Hey, hey wait a minute. Wait, where are you going?
>
> MARLIN: It's over Dory, we were too late. Nemo's gone and I'm going home now.
>
> DORY: No, no, you can't! Stop! Please don't go away, please? No one's ever stuck with me so long before. And if you leave, if you leave—I, I remember things better with you. I do, look, P. Sherman, 42, 42 . . . I remember it, I do, it's there, I know it is, because when I look at you, I can feel it, and I look at you and I'm—home. I don't want that to go away. I don't want to forget.
>
> MARLIN: I'm sorry, Dory, but I do.

Marlin ignores Dory's plea and swims on. Alone, confused, and swimming in circles, Dory encounters Nemo, who was, after all, just *pretending* to be dead to escape his fate as the pet of the dentist's sadistic niece, Darla. "Nemo. That's a nice name!" she says, with no recognition that she just traveled half the ocean to find him. Later, Dory does have a flash of lucidity—remembering Nemo and pushing him on to find his father.

In *Finding Nemo,* short-term memory loss is challenging but not debilitating when one is surrounded by supportive friends. In fact, Dory is an indispensable part of the team here, and Nemo would not have been found without her. Her flash of lucidity, in which she remembers that she was looking for Nemo, is a realistic and temporary flash, unlike the fantasy of extended lucidity in *The Notebook.* By the end of *Finding Nemo,* Dory has once again forgotten Nemo's name. The viewer is invited to identify with Dory as *more* than her disability. She has a complex personality. She is courageous and naïve at the same time. Although her future is not imagined in the film, she clearly has a valued place in the clownfish family. She's ready for a sequel.

The humans in *Finding Nemo* are marked with age—the dentist, for example, has gray hair. The absence of age markings on the fish does not make them ageless—they are marked with perky energy and the ages of the voices of the actors who play them—a healthy, early middle age, the wide window of "parenthood." But the simple fact that these are fish allows us to set aside our fears of aging and age-related memory loss long enough to identify with a main character with "short-term memory loss" whose experiences parallel those of so many older adults. Dory has short-term memory loss. She has no personality changes, no hallucinations, no long-term memory loss, no loss of physical function. But Dory gives us a way to start seeing people with memory loss as experiencing more than just loss.

When I sat down to write about *Nemo,* the dialogue poured out of my fingertips. Like my son, Ben, I had memorized every line. Ben has since moved beyond *Nemo.* His latest favorite is a double DVD collection of *Super Friends* episodes featuring Wonder Woman, Superman, Batman and Robin, Aquaman, and the Wonder Twins (and their space monkey, Gleek) that I watched religiously as a child. I watched it on television—DVDs had not been invented yet. When Ben and I share popcorn side by side on the couch, I know before it happens that Sinbad the Space Pirate will steal the loot from Easter Island, in a final, evil act before the Super Friends figure out how to defeat him. (Note to my eventual caregivers: I might show some physical response to the Super Friends, but I much prefer *Nemo.*)

In an ad campaign from 2005, the Alzheimer's Association took a "Nemo"-like approach to memory loss. The "Maintain Your Brain" ad campaign did not feature any older adults. In one image, a young, smiling African American woman is speed walking across the tall, narrow space of the ad. "Think Fast" appears multiple times on a banner behind her. The image is slightly blurred, as though she's walking so fast the camera can barely catch her. The effect is compounded by the fact that she's walking to the left and we read to the right—making our eyes zigzag to take in the image. "Think Fast" is the only ad in this series that features a person. Other ads include "Think Round," with a close-up shot of a plate full of plump blueberries, and "Think Square," with a close-up of freshly sharpened pencil about to fill in 22 down of a crossword puzzle. These ads take a "Nemo" approach—memory loss and dementia are everyone's (every species?) concern, not just older adults'. We should *all* be exercising our brains, our bodies, and our minds. The ads tell us that we don't need to *see* older adults to understand that memory loss is a problem we should all address.

The 2007 advertising push by the Alzheimer's Association continued this train of thought. The $8 million campaign took a two-pronged approach. First, the association made an effort to move beyond public service announcements, adopting a strategy similar to the traditional media blitz by buying space in major magazines such as *Newsweek, Parade,* and *Time* and online at aol.com, msn.com, oprah.com, and prevention.com. The ads featured an abstract image of a person (unreadable for age, ethnicity, or gender). Text, writ large, appeared on the bottom half of the image, with one word singled out for emphasis. There were three varieties. The first stated: "Many Alzheimer's sufferers will slowly lose control of their bodies. They need you to MOVE their cause forward." The second stated: "Someone suffering from Alzheimer's will lose the ability to form thoughts, remember simple words, and ultimately communicate. You can be their VOICE." Finally, the third ad in this campaign stated: "As their brains continue to shrink people with Alzheimer's will feel trapped in their own minds. They need you to OPEN everyone else's." The campaign emphasizes the emergency of Alzheimer's to urge the general public toward committed action. This is clearly a very good thing. Yet somehow, the ads also insinuate something that can seem both demeaning and frightening to the many people in the early stages of memory loss—that people with Alzheimer's are incapable of advocating for themselves.

The second prong of the 2007 public relations campaign featured "Alzheimer's champions," celebrities who put their image, charm, and stories behind the cause. The idea was that celebrity champions would pique the interest of major television shows—and it worked. According to public relations director Mary Schwartz, the campaign landed the Alzheimer's Association slots on *The View, The Martha Stewart Show,* and *Today.* In the Web images, the stars appear in relative close-up, in purple T-shirts with one of the three key words of the campaign—MOVE (toward a cure), OPEN (your eyes), VOICE (your opinion)—written on them. Peter Gallagher, Olympia Dukakis, Vivica Fox, "Dear" Abby, Brent Spiner, Dick Van Dyke, Kate Burton, Steven Pasquale, Ricki Lake, David Hyde Pierce, Shelley Fabares, Victor Garber, Lea Thompson, Jack Ford, Kate Mulgrew, Dominic Chianese, Natalie Morales, Bob Goen, Sarah Polley, Tracie Thoms, Jean Smart, and Phyllis George are the human celebrities. The gallery of photos on the Web site also features Diamond Jim, the 2007 Westminster Dog Show–winning English springer spaniel, with a purple bandana around his neck. News releases explain that Diamond Jim is a pet therapy dog for people with dementia. The video that accompanies the photo gallery on the alz.org Web site shows the stars posing for their photos and shares short snippets of interviews with each in which they share their personal experience with the disease. Alzheimer's has affected their mothers, fathers, grandfathers, stepfathers, and friends. Traci Thoms says, "It can hit people as early as their 30s. I think if more people knew that, they'd join the fight." The copy of the paid ad with the MOVE slogan likewise emphasizes the early-onset form of Alzheimer's. The smaller type reads "More than 250,000 people under 65 won't be able to stop the progression of Alzheimer's. Maybe you will."

Will including young, celebrity spokespersons in the promotional campaign and understanding that dementia can strike "young" people make more people join the cause? Knowing the depth and mechanisms of ageism in the United States, I think the answer is probably "yes." Unlike *Nemo* and the other films in which older people were missing from the memory loss plots, the 2007 celebrity champions campaign did feature older men and women. Abby, Dominic Chianese, Dick Van Dyke, and Olympia Dukakis wear their age beautifully. The 2007 campaign, paid or unpaid, just didn't feature any older men and women with dementia. As of this writing, the Alzheimer's Association has never featured a person with the disease in a national advertising campaign. Its public relations team does have an extensive list of spokespeople with dementia and their caregivers whom it connects with reporters doing stories about the disease experience. But in the paid advertisements and high-profile celebrity campaign, the images are cleansed of dementia. This is tricky territory, and in some ways, the association is damned if it does and damned if it doesn't. The disability rights movement has sharply criticized the "poster child" approach to disease awareness campaigns. Such campaigns hold up a person with a disease or disability as an object to be pitied. On the other hand, a spokesperson with dementia who was more than an object of pity, one who passionately spoke for him- or herself, for example, might leave the public saying, "Well, that disease isn't so bad."

The Alzheimer's Association has a challenging line to walk. How does it try to raise awareness among the general population, most of whom have heard of Alzheimer's but few of whom know much about it, and get out the message that there is an association to support those with the disease? How does it address the needs and acknowledge the abilities of people diagnosed before age 65? How does it cut through ageism and fear of dementia to create empathy without making people with dementia seem completely helpless? The association is starting to address this quandary—of how to be a voice for the many thousands of people being diagnosed earlier while they are still able to live normal lives, of how to compete with the constantly sounding alarm bells in our 24-hour news cycle, in which the terror alert level seems stuck on red. In 2007, the association created a place on the national board for someone with dementia. As the biggest generation in our history advances toward the age of dementia, this quandary will only get trickier.

7

All of the Above

Denny Crane as the Clown of Dementia

❧ BRAD CHASE: You're now becoming something to parody. . . . You're
a complete joke. . . . I adore you, but it hurts to see you deteriorating into a . . .
DENNY CRANE: Get the hell out of my office.

Boston Legal

William Shatner, barrel chested and slightly bloated, bursts through the doors of a conference room. "Denny Crane!" he declares and waits, politely, for his audience of fellow attorneys to absorb the shock and awe of the moment. Crane is a named partner in the fictional Boston law firm of Crane, Pool, and Schmidt on ABC's *Boston Legal,* which premiered October 3, 2004.

Boston Legal revolves around several core characters. Denny Crane (Shatner) is a living, legal legend. He is outrageous in all respects; in his courtroom antics, sexual appetite, flexible ethics, and his conservative politics, which includes a rabid love of guns (which always seem to be loaded). Crane's doppelgänger is Alan Shore (James Spader), an attorney some 20 years his junior, and yet his equal in outrageousness. Other attorneys, like Shirley Schmidt (Candice Bergen) and Brad Chase (Mark Valley), have been dispatched to "control" Denny. Shore and Crane bond in a mission to thwart their partners at every turn.

I had heard that *Boston Legal* addressed dementia but was unprepared for just how deeply it ran as a theme. Initially, I caught a few episodes from the 2007 season. Intrigued, I ordered the disc sets of seasons 1 and 2 and started watching. I was incredulous. This was some of the best imagery of memory loss I'd seen in mass media. Almost the entire first season is perched on the precarious line between sanity and insanity. In the opening scene of the first episode, Edwin Poole (another named partner) arrives for a meeting without pants. "Demagnetize his parking pass," says Crane coldly after Poole is hauled away by paramedics. "I know when a man is gone." But does he? Is *he?*

Boston Legal gives us lawyers on the verge of snapping as they are pushed to the limits of sanity, ethics, morality, and billable hours. Crane begins the series convinced he has Alzheimer's. His colleagues agree. "The partners will not allow you to dismantle [the firm] with your buffoonery!" scolds Paul Lewiston, an unnamed and uptight partner played with delicious rigidity by René Auberjonois. Denny suspects that there might be something wrong with him but steadfastly refuses to let them see him sweat. In between Tourette-like outbursts on the topics of guns, sex, and breakfast cereals ("Cuckoo for Cocoa Puffs," he mutters under his breath in one scene in "Schmidt Happens" [season 1, episode 11]), Denny insists on his dignity and relevance. Alan Shore, who sees Crane for all that he is, lovingly helps him cover his tracks while holding his feet to the fire.

It might sound crazy, but I believe that a team of Dory, the little blue fish from *Finding Nemo,* and Denny Crane, at least as he appears in the first season of *Boston Legal,* could help usher us into a new mainstream cultural understanding of memory loss. This new conception is one in which people with memory loss are a vital part of plot and family and in which seeming opposites—growth/loss, humor/tragedy, wisdom/foolishness, disease/vitality—live as equals.

Crane embodies all these contradictions. In "Still Crazy after All These Years," the second episode in the first season, Brad Chase flatly tells Denny what's happening around him. Brad was brought in to "manage" Denny and save the firm from embarrassment. "You're now becoming something to parody," says Brad. "You're a complete joke . . . I adore you, but it hurts to see you deteriorating into a . . ." "Get the hell out of my office," snaps Denny. Denny might entertain his own fears, but he won't entertain the doubts of others—unless he can use those doubts to his advantage.

Later in the same episode, the partners decide to let Denny argue a case by himself—in the hope that he will humiliate himself so badly that he'll finally have the wisdom to retire. As Denny enters the courtroom, the background music is a strong bass beat with the lyrics "Bring it on." Crane redeems himself and wins the day with a closing that seems both crazy and purposeful. When Brad Chase comes in to congratulate him, Crane says, "I don't need your praise. . . . I want your respect! I'm a senior partner. Respect goes with the job. Not to mention I've earned it. Don't you think I feel the wagons circling?"

In this same episode, Crane confronts his partner Paul. "I'm still a good lawyer," he insists. "Yes. You are," confirms Paul, who then recalls how Muhammad Ali got creamed in his last fight. "The tragedy that night, Denny, wasn't that he couldn't still box. He could. The tragedy was that he still thought he was Ali. You're still a good lawyer, my friend. You're just not Denny Crane."

At the end of "An Eye for an Eye" (season 1, episode 5), Denny Crane and Alan Shore share a scotch in a jail cell after Crane has been cited for contempt of court. Alan compliments Denny on his theatrical closing that earned him a mistrial to the advantage of their client.

DENNY: I wasn't clever. I forgot.

ALAN: I beg your pardon?

DENNY: I stood up, armed with all the facts of our client's billing practices, and . . . I went blank in front of the jury. I couldn't remember a damn thing.

ALAN: Well, that can happen sometimes.

DENNY: You once said you suspected I had Alzheimer's. How does a person know?

ALAN: Well, there's no exact diagnostic—they can do certain tests. Denny, you may have gone up on an opening, but to recover like that and go for a mistrial—that's evidence of a man thinking quickly on his feet.

DENNY: I want to take the test.

The episode closes on this quiet, serious note, as Alan rubs Denny's shoulders to comfort him. Denny is no buffoon here. He is like countless others whose heartbeat races when they speak the word—"Alzheimer's"—out loud.

In the sixth episode of season 1 ("Truth Be Told"), Denny goes to the doctor. He is pure peacock. But we aren't quite sure what the bright colors are hiding.

DOCTOR: Now, I'm going to ask you a series of . . .

DENNY: Denny Crane!

DOCTOR: Why did you just say that?

DENNY: Well, isn't that how you guys usually begin a mental-status examination, by determining if the subject knows his own name?

DOCTOR: Well, yes.

DENNY: Denny Crane.

DOCTOR: Got it. And who am I, Mr. Crane?

DENNY: (*reading his nametag*) You are Doctor Thomas H. Lee, neurologist.

DOCTOR: Good. Can you tell me what day of the week this is?

DENNY: Monday. And a particularly crisp and beautiful one, too, I might add.

DOCTOR: Good. And who is the current president of the United States?

DENNY: That would be Ernest Borgnine.

(*There is a pause.*)

DENNY: Ah. I'll bet you get lunatics in here everyday that—that say that stuff for real, right? The current president of the United States is George Walker Bush, son to George Herbert Walker Bush, whose father was the late United States Senator Prescott Bush, who, as an undergraduate at Yale, once wrestled my father in the nude. But that's a story for another day. Let's stick to the issues at hand.

He ends with his typical exclamation point, a strong, confident affirmation of who he is: "Denny Crane."

The rest of the episode could be a promotional video for the Alzheimer's Association's "Maintain Your Brain" program. Denny enthusiastically exercises his brain. He preaches to his partners about the benefits of keeping yourself challenged. When Paul pays him a visit to chide him about not bringing enough money to the firm, Denny encourages him to do crossword puzzles. Another colleague catches him on the computer. "Have you ever used a computer before?" she asks. "An entirely new experience!" he says in delight. Later, Paul again confronts Denny about this new, bizarre behavior.

PAUL: Denny, I'm worried about you. You're speaking French to the messengers. You've got crosswords spread out all over the conference tables. You walk into a reception, hijack one of Sally Heep's clients, actually have a meeting with him in your office!—did you even know what his case was about?

DENNY: I took that test the other day. The one where they ask you a bunch of questions to see if you've turned into an imbecile. Then they do a scan of your brain. You know what they found out? That I have a lot of blue and yellow and red stuff colliding up there. The damn MRI photo looks like a hurricane. I don't remember what was the good color and what was the bad color, but the point is this. They discovered that I remember some things, and I forget others.

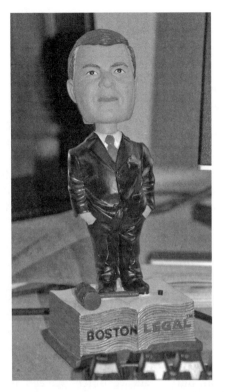

My Denny Crane "bobble-head" sits by my computer. Photo by Anne Basting.

(*There is a pause; he makes a gesture with an open mouth and outstretched arms that says, ironically, "Imagine that!"*)

And that's the way it's going to be.

It turns out that Denny did know what Sally Heep's client's case was about and that he manipulated both the client and defendants into a settlement and a multimillion-dollar contract for their future legal work. "So don't you worry too much, Paul, about Denny Crane," he says.

Denny refuses pity. He insists on respect. He is allergic to apology. He uses his "condition" to keep people guessing. "Every once in a while, just to keep 'em guessing, I stick a cigar in my ear," he says in episode 9 of season 1. He is a poster child for living in the moment, fully committed to one's convictions, no matter how outrageous. In a quiet moment over scotch at the end of episode 1 of season one, Alan asks Denny, "Are you scared?" Denny responds, "The only thing to be scared of, son, is tomorrow. I don't live for tomorrow. Never saw the fun in it." Crane also refuses the label "Alzheimer's." Instead, he calls his malady "mad cow," as if to mock it, himself, and the medical framework for what is happening to him. He ridicules his condition: "May I express a thought? I so rarely get one," he says in episode 8.

Denny Crane is *every* storyline on memory loss swirling about in the body of one man. This is a remarkably complex achievement for prime-time television. The usual in mainstream stories is simplicity. Good or bad. Comic or tragic. Stories that live in the gray area between these polarities tend to land in the ghetto of independent film and/or PBS, where the audience numbers are much smaller. It proved difficult to sustain the complexity and dynamism of Denny Crane's wrestling with Alzheimer's past the first season. There are moments in subsequent shows in which Denny shines, but nothing like the manifesto of the first season. He slips into progressively sillier scenarios (shooting a fish and a duck in two separate shows).

But even in the 2007 season, Crane stands as a model for the struggle of older men and women, regardless of their cognitive health, to find a reason for being. As Crane says to Shirley Schmidt after she admonishes him for shooting the duck: "Shirley, you're a beautiful woman—smart, still relevant, really. But you're old. You're closing in on the end. Not as fast as I am, but . . . ah, we're rich. We certainly don't need to work, but we do so, not only because we love it, but because we're desperate for distraction—like running around shooting a shotgun. It can be more fun than sitting in your office acting your age."

Part Three

MOVING THROUGH FEAR

Stories about Dementia That Inspire Hope

> ❧ With the past as past, I have nothing to do; nor with the future as future. I live now.
>
> Ralph Waldo Emerson

The week after Roger was diagnosed with dementia, he fell into depression. "We were both very scared," said his wife, Rocille. And then, miraculously, an article appeared in their hometown paper about a support group starting up for people in the early stages of memory loss. "I couldn't believe it," said Rocille. "I called immediately, talked to the facilitator, and she told me she had 10 members now and she was going to take only three more. So we made an appointment immediately to see her." The group made all the difference in the world. Roger found strength in numbers. "There's nobody there that's uppity-uppity," he said. "It's all just people my age." Rocille took hope in Roger's newfound confidence. "I must tell you he was a different person completely," she said. "He came home that day with a big smile on this face. He was with people who he knew had similar problems to him and yet they were coping, and it gave him hope."

After 2 weeks in the program, Roger tested his mettle. His colleagues on a county committee were talking about the article and the new support group. He told them that it was a great program—and that he was a member. "I was so proud of him," said Rocille, "because one of the things I've learned is that one of the biggest problems is getting the person accepted." Roger started telling everybody. They've been lucky—they have been embraced by friends and family. "The only thing I notice is that people don't like to talk about it," said Roger.

By moving through our fears, we can find hope—hope that embraces the person as he or she is rather than looking solely to the future (for a cure) or the past (exalting who the person *was*). In the following

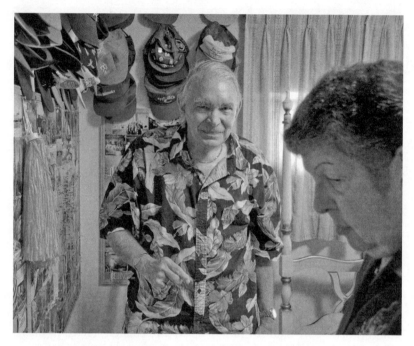

Roger McConnell. Photo by www.jimherrington.com.

chapters, I profile 10 different approaches to moving through fear to find hope in the moment of dementia, be it early, middle, or late stage. These chapters tell the stories of the people who created the programs and of people who found hope and meaning in them. These programs don't shy away from the serious challenges dementia can raise. Loss is a core part of the experience of dementia. But these programs also find value and meaning in human connection in the present moment. In these stories, people find each other through the simple grasping of hands, the movement of a paintbrush, the asking of questions, and the patient listening for answers—in whatever way they come.

Alzheimer's is not only a disease of the mind but also of the environment. We live in a culture that prizes independence and the rugged individual capable of doing for him- or herself. We live in a time when the markings of age are a source of embarrassment and a sign of a lack of power (or the will and financial means to remove them). A youthful appearance has become the ultimate consumer product. "Antiaging" motifs decorate moisturizer labels and the business cards of doctors alike.

And yet our time is also one in which more people than ever are living long, healthy lives. And more people than ever are experiencing dementia.

The 10 programs I profile in this section all take a step toward redefining the cultural environment of dementia and memory loss. They deemphasize the *give* in caregiving and instead stress the extent to which it is a reciprocal partnership. There is something to be learned, gifts to be exchanged, in every partnership. In the introduction to part 1, I described the fears attached to the experience of dementia; by far the most common is the fear of being a burden. We fear becoming a burden because we imagine that caregivers give and people with dementia take and take and take until there is nothing left to give—financially, physically, or emotionally. In the programs I profile here, people with dementia are seen as having a great deal to offer those who support their care, including audiences of people whom they'll never meet—the general public. In these profiles, we find people who happen to have dementia teaching young adults about what is important in life. We hear their voices and original lyrics on professional recordings. We see them capturing the world around them in photographs. We see them dancing to original choreography. We read their original stories—both fiction and nonfiction. We become aware that they provide positive models for our own old age. People with dementia offer all of us their vision of the world in images, movements, songs, stories, and phrases. It is a vision both complex and contradictory at times, ranging from the lifting energy of humor to the ache of despair. It is a vision that can teach us about resiliency and the human drive for meaning and recognition regardless of disability. It is a vision that can compel us to reexamine our care practices, our long-term care policies, our attitudes toward aging and dementia.

The programs I outline emphasize the value of being in the present moment.

They emphasize memory as relational, as existing between people, not as belonging to one person or another.

They offset our fears of meaninglessness by filling that void with meaning and providing the tools for making it.

The use of fear in marketing grabs our attention. But it can also invite despair and fuel stigma. Canny marketing approaches, storytelling, and the creation of programs that inspire action and hope for meaningful human connection might bring us closer to a world in which the estimated five million people with dementia today, and their 19 million friends and family, might find the strength to carry on. As we wait for scientists to bring us a cure, or, at the very least, clear steps for prevention, programs like these begin to cure the cultural context in which we experience dementia.

8

StoryCorps and the
Memory Loss Initiative

❧ I was diagnosed in 2004 with Alzheimer's. I was 50. A friend of mine
sent me an e-mail right after my diagnosis, she said this is terrible,
this isn't fair, this is a horrible thing. And I wrote back to her and I
said, well, it's not that bad. It's not like you're in pain all the time.
But it takes a toll on our family because I know that when they see
my failing they get really sad and they don't like to see that. I wish
they would try to understand that I may be a little different—there
is a time there where I will forget everybody's name. But inside, I'm
still here, I'm still me. Inside I'm thinking how much fun I'm having
with them, and I as much as possible would like to be treated as I
had been treated before.

Charles Jackson

Asking a question and listening to the response—really listening—demands time, focus, attention, and an acknowledgment that the person
is worthy of being heard. Listening—really listening—is a lost art. But
it's a simple concept. And it is the core of StoryCorps.

Wrapped around that core is one of the fastest-growing nonprofit organizations in the country. StoryCorps is a national oral history project
that encourages everyday people to share the stories of their lives. A
StoryCorps interview is a son asking his mother about her childhood. It
is a young woman asking her grandfather about his first love. It is a
couple reminiscing about their first or their fiftieth wedding anniversary. When you set out for your StoryCorps experience, a well-trained
facilitator greets you at one of the StoryCorps booths: a sumptuously
designed permanent booth in New York City; semipermanent story
booths in various locations; and mobile booths inside of two, soundproof Airstream trailers that crisscross the country. No doubt, by the
time you read this, there will be many more.

I visited the StoryCorps booth in Grand Central Station in New York City, in 2006. That majestic building itself is an adventure, with the rhythmic rushing of commuters dodging tourists stopped and staring slack jawed up at the domed ceiling. I joined the flow of traffic and went to the central information booth, with its old-fashioned clock, and asked directions to the StoryCorps booth. They guided me in detail, and, surprisingly, slowly enough for me to hear and remember. I wound my way back toward the tracks, turned a corner, and came upon an orange and silver booth. It was compact and luminous. A friendly facilitator welcomed me. I was supposed to have met a friend, but like many New Yorkers, he got swept away by meetings. One of the StoryCorps facilitators would have to stand in and ask me meaningful questions about my life. I ducked into the soundproof chamber, and the frenetic world of Grand Central disappeared. I sat down in front of an enormous microphone, knee to knee with the facilitator and enveloped by the soft light, warm colors, and round lines of the booth. "What kind of childhood did you have?" she asked. I'd never thought about that. What kind of childhood *did* I have? And so it began.

A StoryCorps interview is a moving experience. The size and quality of the microphone acts as an angel on your shoulder, compelling you set aside the "flexible" truths of our everyday conversations and to dredge up stories, images, and thoughts with more freshness and honesty than you might otherwise. The coziness and sumptuous design of the booth, as well as the earnest idealism of the StoryCorps staff, encourages you to leave your cynicism at the door. I was here to be heard, possibly for generations to come.

After the interview, the StoryCorps facilitator handed me a disc of the interview to keep and share as I like. The stories I told about my grandmother will be great to share with my own grandchildren. I also gave permission for StoryCorps to use the interview however it might like (possibly cutting it for public radio) and to send a copy to the Library of Congress's American Folklife Center. Excerpts of a slim percentage of the over 10,000 interviews StoryCorps has facilitated since 2003 are edited and broadcast on National Public Radio as part of *Morning Edition.* StoryCorps invites you to open yourself to the story-sharing experience, and then, through its connections with National Public Radio and the Library of Congress, weaves your story into the fabric of American history.

The concept for StoryCorps was a bold dream, built on the shoulders of the Federal Writers Project of the 1930s. StoryCorps founder David Isay is an accomplished radio documentarian whose striking works on the residents of ghettos, flophouses, and prisons have won multiple awards. The idea for StoryCorps grew out of Isay's belief that documentary can foster positive change in people's lives, particularly those who live where justice is scarce, when their stories are told truthfully, respectfully, and with stunning sound quality. Perhaps the MacArthur Fellowship he received in 2000 enabled him to take the next big step: to realize a project that would encourage Americans to be better listeners and to help us recognize the dignity and strength in neighbors we've never met.

In 2006, StoryCorps began working with a team of advisors to make the StoryCorps experience accessible to people with memory loss. I was one of them. It was a natural next step for StoryCorps. People of all ages visit the booth, but it has a special draw for those who feel their stories might soon be lost to age or illness. In the first year of what we called the Memory Loss Initiative (MLI), we aimed to educate the StoryCorps staff about the experience of memory loss, adapt the StoryCorps materials and guidelines for those with memory loss, promote the StoryCorps experience so that people with memory loss knew that it was open to them, and evaluate the StoryCorps experience for visitors who came to the booth as part of the MLI. The goal was to conduct a modest 40 interviews with people with memory loss.

The StoryCorps facilitators and general staff are an inspiring group. They are broadly diverse in age and economic and ethnic background. The earn very little, but they thrive on the mission and experience. The facilitators dutifully responded to surveys about their understanding of and attitudes toward dementia both before and after MLI training in July 2006. According to the surveys, basic training about memory loss led to some significant shifts. The surveys detected significant increases in their comfort level about interacting with people with dementia, their understanding of how to communicate with people with dementia, and their perception that one *can* connect with people with dementia. The surveys also suggested that the staff came away from the training with greater general knowledge about dementia and memory loss.

To help lay the groundwork for successful interviews, the StoryCorps MLI advisory group put together a list of interview tips. People *without* memory loss can be frustrating to people *with* memory loss. These tips were designed to help reduce that frustration. In general, interviews are most successful if people shed their expectations of oral histories filled with facts and figures. MLI interviews are more focused on the emotional exchange between those who visit the booth. Sometimes, the most powerful part of an interview is the capturing of the person's voice in a professional-quality recording. The MLI interview tips are good guidelines for everyday conversation but are particularly helpful for communicating with people who have cognitive challenges:

Use short sentences. Try not to combine two ideas. For example, it's best to ask, "How did it feel growing up during the Depression?" and then, later, follow up with "Did you feel poor?" rather than combining the two thoughts.

Speak at a normal rate—not too slow but not too fast.

Keep in mind that it might take a while for someone to process a question or come up with an answer. Be patient. Don't follow up with another question right away.

A little prompting may be necessary. It may be helpful to provide some information before you ask a question. For example, you might say, "I know you and Dad met at a school dance. I wonder how you felt when you first saw him."

You might have to phrase the same question a number of different ways before a person understands it. Here is an example: "Tell me about your brother, John." "You and your brother John are so close now. Why do you think that's the case?" "It seems as if your brother John has always been your favorite brother. Why do you think that is?"

Don't hesitate to share some of your own stories about the storyteller with him or her during the interview. Those stories often spark a memory or just delight the person.

Be general when you ask a question. Instead of asking about the "happiest" or "hardest" times in the person's life, ask about "happy times" or "hard times."

If someone goes off topic, go with him. Sometimes the best conversations happen this way. You can always redirect the person to your original question later.

Assure the storyteller that it's okay to ask for clarification. It's okay to say, "I don't remember." You can simply rephrase a question or ask a new question and return to the topic later.

Be aware that the interview experience might evoke some of your own emotions—emotions you may not have realized were so close to the surface. It will probably bring you much joy, but it also can also evoke feelings of loss or sorrow.

Enjoy the opportunity to share the stories, thoughts, and emotional closeness that comes with this experience.

As of this writing, five MLI interviews have played on NPR. Two of them in particular are textbook examples of good interviewing and tell full, complicated stories of memory loss that garner tremendous empathy. The national reach and emotional power of these stories go a long way toward helping ease the stigma of memory loss. These two interviews received scores of e-mail responses from listeners of NPR's *Morning Edition*. In one interview, played for Valentine's Day in 2007, an Arkansas couple, Bob and JoAnn Chew, talk about both the challenges of her Alzheimer's and their deep love for each other. The interview flashes from lighthearted to deeply emotional and back again. The diagnosis of Alzheimer's has clearly shaken them both. But JoAnn's quick and infectious giggle and Bob's steady, affirming voice also reveal their inner strength. For example, JoAnn tells the story of the limited choices for women when she was growing up. Her father told her she could go to college if she took home economics (to learn to be somebody's wife) or secretarial training. She chose home economics and became a wonderful cook.

BOB: Are you still cooking today?

JOANN: Not today, I have up to this point. But I have Alzheimer's, the beginning of it, so I hear. And my doctor told me he did not want me to cook. And that was music to my ears!

BOB: (*laughing*) Who is doing all the cooking?

JOANN: (*laughing*) This fellow across from me here. And he's turned out to be quite a professional, too!

Later, Bob and JoAnn get more serious. Bob asks her if she gets down about her diagnosis:

JOANN: A little bit . . . a little bit. (*pause*) A big bit.

BOB: A big bit.

JOANN: I'm sad.

BOB: What's making you sad?

JOANN: Just not having control of everything, my thoughts and my actions. And I don't think it's fair to you either.

BOB: You know I'm going to take care of you, don't you?

> JOANN: I know, but you could have some little chick 10 years younger that
>   you could be running around with.
> BOB: But I have my princess right here.
> JOANN: Oh, you're wonderful . . .

In another StoryCorps interview that played on NPR's *Morning Edition,* Ken Morganstern was interviewed by his daughters, Priya Morganstern and Bhavani Jaroff. They don't directly address Ken's memory loss. Instead, they talk about Ken meeting his wife and their mother. They talk about their family and the rhythm of his days. They talk about what they mean to each other.

> PRIYA: What's your life like now, Dad?
> KEN: It's a wonderful life. I get up in the morning, go to sleep at night, and
>   in between eat three meals.
> (*They all laugh.*)
> KEN: What's wrong with that?
> (*They all laugh.*)
> PRIYA: It's a nice thing that it's so easy to make you happy, Dad.
> KEN: I'm very much like my father; he was an easy-going guy. People used
>   to call him "Happy Harry." And I have a lot of his characteristics, I think.
> PRIYA: Do you have any regrets, Dad?
> KEN: I'm sitting here thinking I have no regrets on anything. The impor-
>   tant thing is I have a family I love and they are loving people. That's the
>   biggest thing you can leave as a . . . a . . . a . . .
> PRIYA: Legacy.
> KEN: A legacy, yeah.
> PRIYA: I want to tell you, Dad, that I've always considered you my guru and
>   teacher.
> BHAVANI: I would say the same. You've been a role model for all of your
>   family. People are constantly saying to us how lucky you are to have all
>   of us, and I turn to them and I say: we are because of him. You've cre-
>   ated such love around you and we want to be with you.
> KEN: Thank you, honey. That's awfully nice to hear.
> PRIYA: It's the truth.
> BHAVANI: We love you, Dad.

The e-mails that poured in to *Morning Edition* in response to these two clips were as moving as the stories themselves. They came from older couples who found inspiration in the Chews. They came from a young

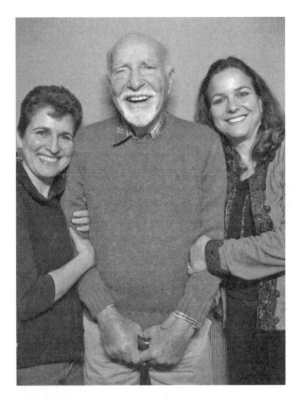

Ken Morganstern with daughters Priya and Bhavani. Photo courtesy of StoryCorps (www.storycorps.net).

woman, with no experience with dementia, who hoped that her new marriage would blossom and endure like the Chews'. They came from adult sons and daughters who empathized with and admired the Morgansterns.

In December 2006, Dina Zempsky joined StoryCorps as the coordinator of the MLI project. Zempsky, a certified geriatric social worker based in Brooklyn, is a blend of infinite patience and ebullient passion. Zempsky preinterviews every person who marks "memory loss initiative" on the online or 800-number reservation system to help him or her understand the mission of the project. She guided the MLI toward a near tripling of its original, first-year goal of 40 interviews in New York and Milwaukee to 110 interviews nationwide and set the goal for the subsequent 3 years of the initiative at over 400 interviews a year. When I asked her if she felt like the program was having an impact, she said:

Oh, I really do. The hope for the clips that are broadcast are enormous. We need them to educate people about how much dementia we have in this country, and to start thinking about how we're going to take care of these folks. We need people to think about this early stage a little differently—as a place where people can have some creativity and peace in their lives.

In the first pilot year of the MLI in 2006, StoryCorps set out to learn about how to improve the process for those with memory loss. University of Wisconsin Milwaukee Center on Age and Community (CAC) scholar Marie Savundranayagam helped design a study that included phone interviews with the person with memory loss and the interviewer up to 10 days after their StoryCorps experience. CAC researcher Lorna Dilley also called again up to 3 months later to see if there was any lasting effect. The response was overwhelmingly positive. One hundred percent of the people with memory loss and 100 percent of the friends or family interviewers said they would recommend the experience to others. After 3 months, 53 percent of family or friend interviewers said the StoryCorps experience had enabled them to have more meaningful conversations, and 76 percent said they had used the CD. Several themes emerged in the evaluations of StoryCorps. The experience helped people appreciate the beauty of the present moment. The StoryCorps facilitators, trained to model attention and respect, made an enormous difference. One person said of her facilitator that she "was just a beautiful young woman—I mean she really—she had a major impact on us. The fact that she's involved in that type of work, and just seems to enjoy it so much, it was very touching. And she seemed very affected by the interview herself. I mean when we were laughing, she was hysterical! She had tears rolling down her face and then at the end when my father [got] kind of, you know, pretty emotional and sentimental, she had tears in her eyes, and you know, it just seemed like she's doing something she loves. So that was very positive."

The evaluations also showed that the StoryCorps experience enabled people to raise new issues, clarify existing issues, and feel as though they were leaving a legacy to future generations. The only negative responses were that some participants felt odd about talking into such a large microphone and some were haunted by thoughts that they could have done better if they had another chance.

Zempsky says this feeling, that the participants failed in some way, is one she hears about and tries to stamp out several times a day. People hear the clips on NPR and think that they need to come in with a charming or gut-wrenching, linear, and tightly told story. "But the mission isn't a linear interview. If that happens, that's great, but it's not necessary," said Zempsky. She likes to use one interview in particular as an example. StoryCorps facilitators went out to do a series of "door-to-door" interviews, in which they take the equipment out to particular sites. At an adult day program in New York, they interviewed a man named Mel. "Mel had one story," said Zempsky, "which he repeated over and over again for 40 minutes. It made the facilitators a little anxious. But he was so happy. I use this as an example to show people that it's not about getting it right. This is a chance for them to use their 40 minutes to say whatever they want to say."

I listened to the clip the StoryCorps production team made to share Mel's story at conferences. He tells a story about playing baseball in his half-Jewish, half-Italian neighborhood as a kid and about being asked to play the harmonica (that his father gave him) at a neighbor's party. He couldn't have been more proud. Mel even brought his harmonica into the booth. "Do you have any requests?" he asks. "Play 'The Merry Widow,'" says social worker Lindsay Goldman on the tape. "That was my mother's favorite!" he says, surprised that she would know this. His breathy and lively rendition of the song leaves you yearning for more—of him, of the song, of your parents, your grandparents, and of StoryCorps.

9

Memory Bridge

❧ "Do you have any children?" Jessica, herself a teenaged mom, asks.
"Love love love love," Annette says, kissing her hand.

www.memorybridge.org

In 2006–7, 344 high school and junior high students befriended 332 residents of dementia care facilities in the greater Chicago area as part of what's called the Chicagoland Memory Bridge Initiative (CMBI). There are some incredible intergenerational programs across the United States. Elders Share the Arts, in New York, engages school-age children and young adults in myriad storytelling and art-making projects in its Generating Community programs across the expanse of the city. St. Ann Center for Intergenerational Care, in Milwaukee, serves older adults and young children in innovative and integrated programming under one roof. Neighbors Growing Together, at Virginia Tech, teaches professionals, conducts research, and provides programming to multiple generations. There is even the Intergenerational School, in Cleveland, a K–8 school receiving national attention from press and the Department of Education for being a model of "spirited citizenship" and "lifelong learning." The school is colocated with a senior center and a chapter of the Alzheimer's Association and features a program in which people with memory loss read to fourth and fifth graders. But even among the nation's shining lights in intergenerational programming, the CMBI breaks ground in sheer numbers and the depth of its curriculum on dementia.

In its inaugural year, the CMBI worked with 270 students ages 10 to 17. Students who take part in the initiative participate in a 12-week program centering on questions that flummox most adults. What is identity? How can people connect across dementia? What can we learn from each other? The after-school program blends science, arts, and service learning. Students learn about the brain and how memory works. They learn how to communicate, particularly with people with memory loss, using the arts as a conduit. Poetry, storytelling, painting, dance, and letter writing are all part of the CMBI toolbox. People in the early stages of dementia visit the classroom to talk with students about what it's like to live with memory loss.

The "buddy visits," however, are the heart of the program. The CMBI staff members match students with a "buddy" at a care facility near their school and prepare the kids to meet their buddies by working with social workers and family members to gather stories and pictures of their buddies. Buddies meet four times over the 12-week period. Memory Bridge founder Michael Verde said he thought the students would bail out when they first saw the pictures of their buddies. He postponed this part of the project as long as possible. But Verde was happily surprised. The meetings with the older buddies only made the kids buy in to the program more deeply. "They bonded," said Verde. The bonding happens on both sides. The buddy visits bring people with dementia back onto the stage of life: "These buddy visits give these older people an audience again," says CMBI director Mary Cohen. "It's like they get a new sense of purpose."

The semester-long after-school program, currently funded by the Illinois Department of Human Services, culminates with the students creating a gift for their buddy based on what they've learned and experienced. Jessica learned that her buddy, Annette, had been a cabaret dancer in her youth. For her final project, Jessica made a mobile with dancers and pictures of the two of them dangling by ribbons so that Annette could make them spin with just the tap of a finger. Figuring out what gift to give your buddy isn't always easy. Franchaun's buddy, Jenny, never spoke with her. Instead, Jenny just stared at the birds in the nursing home's aviary. Perplexed, Franchaun made a scrapbook for Jenny with images of birds and photos of the buddies on various visits. Sharing the gift with Jenny seemed to break the spell, and for the first time, Jenny talked with Franchaun—about the book, the birds, and their time together.

CMBI teacher Darlene Hall, who started with the program in 2005, said that she was deeply impressed by the students' work on their final projects. The assignment challenges students to create a gift that will leave a "memory mark" with their buddies. The first group of students Hall worked with decided to orchestrate a formal, sit-down dinner party for their buddies:

They created an upscale restaurant, with reservations and everything. They had dinner and then they created pictures as place cards—one side was them, the other side was their buddies. Then last year they made vases filled with all these different colored stones and marbles. Some put their pictures in the vases too. The buddies just loved it. The kids also sang a Frank Sinatra song. I told them that if they were going to do that, they needed to practice and they said, "We will—leave it to us." They got up there and they sang their buddies a love song.

Both Cohen and Verde emphasize that their main concern is the quality of the learning experience. What kind of learning happens through this project? "Listening; empathy; understanding of identity and selfhood and their complexities; practical knowledge like how to take the bus to the facility. All of it," says Verde. Stories on the Memory Bridge Web site reveal lessons learned in empathy. In one classroom discussion on empathy, a video of buddy visits revealed a buddy with a tracheostomy. Students were curious. "What's that hole in her neck?" one asked. Students queried the teacher whether it would be rude to ask about it. According to the story on the Web site:

> The teacher ponders this and then asks the kids, "Do you ever get zits?"
> Everyone nods: yes, they do.
> "Well," she says, "how would you like it if somebody asked you about your zits?"
> Their response is swift and unequivocal: They would not like it, not at all.
> "There's your answer," the teacher replies.

Students participating in CMBI aren't just suburban high achievers in search of an experience to write about on college applications. Some of the students' "life maps," created as part of a lesson plan, show a landscape of gangs, homelessness, and immigration nightmares. Some of the skills the students learn in the program and some of the buddy experiences prove deeply useful to these at-risk students. One young man, who had to struggle to cross rival gang territory to get to the program, asked if he could "use what I learned in Memory Bridge when I talk to the old people in my neighborhood." Another student spent several years skipping school, drinking, and hanging out. She finally switched schools and began to excel, owing to her own tenacity and inner strength. Her buddy turned out to be a woman who had had similar troubles, in the same Chicago neighborhoods. The student says of her buddy, Alice,

"She has white curls and a little mouth. Sometimes she doesn't remember who I am but I just tell her that I came to keep her company. Being in Memory Bridge and visiting Alice makes me feel good. It just makes me feel good at heart."

Because CMBI is an after-school program, and students don't have to do it, the program tends to draw kids who are deeply committed. There is an incentive. Chicago public schools require 40 hours of service learning, and CMBI satisfies 32 of those hours. But, says Cohen, "There are kids who are seniors who don't need that much credit, and they do it because they want to. There is this population of kids out there who don't interact with older people and they are just so curious. So we haven't really had any trouble recruiting." Cohen has been surprised by the kind of students who thrive in the program. The "good" students, who focus on getting good grades, tend to get thrown by the unexpected. Take, for example, the woman who didn't like the painting that her buddy had made as a special parting gift. She tore it up in front of her. Cohen said, "This particular girl wasn't phased by it, but some kids who are a little more academically oriented get really upset by something like that and take it personally."

On occasion, CMBI has worked specifically with programs or schools that prepare students for the health and caring fields. Cohen confessed a disappointment with kids who are choosing the health care path. "They seem to have more preconceived notions of care giving and aren't as open to the Memory Bridge experience," she said.

Teachers who participate in CMBI lead 12, 2.5-hour class sessions that meet after school once a week. As an incentive, teachers are paid a small stipend, and they also get professional development credits for their work. CMBI pays for the supplies. Still, it's extra work for the already overworked. What are the benefits for teachers? Hall found the program when her own mother started to experience dementia. "Some friends told me about it and said I should do it to learn more about dementia," she said. "And then I moved and found out my new neighbor had Alzheimer's." I asked her about the commitment on top of her already demanding duties as a Chicago public school teacher. "Oh, it's a commitment for sure!" she said.

> But it gives me a whole different perspective. It's made me realize how important it is to stop and smell the roses. Like now, I'm taking my lunch and relaxing, versus working through it. The smaller things in life really are im-

portant. Even my neighbor—I was with her this weekend. I see how she looks at nature. The things we walk right by, she loves. "Look at the way the leaves blow in the tree," she said, "Look at how blue the sky is"—things we just take for granted. Now I see them.

Where did the program come from? Founder Michael Verde's path to Memory Bridge is full of curves. He's proud of his east Texas heritage and his diverse talents, which include raising pigs, playing football, writing, reading, and studying theology. His studies led him from an MA in literary studies at the University of Iowa to an MA in theology at the University of Durham in England. For several years he taught high school and college English and then found himself in Washington, D.C., working for A Place for Mom, a free advisory service for people looking for guidance through the labyrinth of long-term care. As luck would have it, one of the people he helped provide answers for was Carla Borden, then program and publications manager of the Smithsonian Institution. They began talking about the link between their passions, for Verde, the humanity of people with memory loss (sparked by Michael's grandfather's experience with dementia) and for Borden, the desire to preserve the stories of all Americans as cultural artifacts. Together they forged a series of meetings with advisors from all disciplines, all areas of medical research, and all walks of care practice. The first manifestation of their labor was the creation of an interview guide to help people participate in the Library of Congress's big Veterans History Project, thereby ensuring that veterans with dementia were not excluded from it.

In 2004, Verde and Borden formed Memory Bridge: A Foundation for Cultural Memory. Shortly after, Verde moved to the Chicago area to teach English at the Lake Forest Academy. There he infused his interests into the curriculum by launching the Lake Forest Academy's Alzheimer's and Multicultural Initiative. The initiative formed the roots of what would become the CMBI curriculum. Initially, Verde funded a pilot of the curriculum himself. The State of Illinois sent out some people to watch it in action. Shortly thereafter, the foundation received a subcontract to offer the curriculum on a larger scale. The contract is a stretch for the Department of Human Services in Illinois, but according to Cohen, it was especially taken with how well the program served two at-risk groups: people with dementia and kids unlikely to graduate from high school.

Mary Cohen came to Memory Bridge from the world of online and adult education. But two of her grandparents had dementia. So when colleague Steve Gilbert, who was working with Verde to design the CMBI curriculum, approached Cohen to direct the project, she was open to the idea and embraced the new challenge of working with younger students. When I asked Cohen what she thought was the most powerful aspect of the program, she talked about a new initiative Memory Bridge developed in the summer of 2007. Some students who go through the program bond with their buddies so deeply that they want to repeat it. But thus far, Memory Bridge has preferred to admit students to the CMBI program who have not done it before, which allows more people to participate in it. The staff had been looking for a way to engage alumni. That summer, they put together a program for 11 students called Heart to Heart. Students met with people with early-onset Alzheimer's and people in the early stages of the disease. The youngest was 38 and the oldest was 69. These are people deeply engaged in life, "normal" by all appearances, but forced to sit back because of their cognitive challenges. They told stories of struggling to achieve their dreams, of working hard to get through school, to get the job, to support the family, only to have the disease strip them of it all at a relatively young age. Now what? What mattered to them? The discussions with the students delved deep into the core question of what makes a person. Is it the trappings of one's life? Or the substance of one's being, one's relationships? The people with early-onset dementia "completely changed what these kids thought of themselves and what their purpose in life is," said Cohen. "The kids now say they talk to other people differently because they see there is more to life than these superficial things that they are being acculturated to."

The Memory Bridge Foundation has taken steps beyond providing a curriculum. In the fall of 2007, Verde produced a documentary called *There Is a Bridge,* which profiles a variety of case studies in which people fairly far into the dementia experience connect with those around them through visual arts, validation therapy, and the Memory Bridge curriculum. The film dives deep into the late stages of dementia, an experience we're most accustomed to seeing depicted as tragedy. And there is plenty of sorrow in the film. A dedicated son talks about his longing for just a few more family Sundays with his once vibrant mother. But *There Is a Bridge* insists that we can reach people that the film *The Forgetting* frames as the living dead. "People with dementia," says Verde, "can remind us of aspects of our own humanity that *we* are forgetting."

I met Verde for lunch in a busy, upscale bistro in downtown Chicago in February 2007. He shared big dreams of having the Memory Bridge curriculum take off across the country. I had no doubt his plans would come to fruition. Polished shoes and high heels clicked on the white tile floors, waiters spun around with trays to avoid collisions in the tightly packed dining room of business people enjoying expense-account lunches. I had to lean forward to hear. The room seemed ready to lift up and take flight. This was as far as we could possibly be from the quiet rooms where students held the hands of people with dementia to coax them into communion. Still, as Michael talked, about his faith, about the sources of his inspiration—the writings of Martin Buber, Emmanuel Lévinas, and Stanley Hauerwas—the sounds of the restaurant muted and I was in that room.

> "Sam," she asks him, crouching to eye level. "Do you know the song 'Sentimental Journey'?" As she sings the first line, her eyes tear. Later, she tells me that her grandfather is dying; this is his favorite song.
>
> "Gonna take a sentimental journey," Kate begins.
>
> Sam is now smiling. "Gonna set my mind at ease," he joins in, his voice clear and strong.
>
> "Gonna take a sentimental journey, to renew old memories," they continue together.

To Whom I May Concern

✨ To Whom I May Concern,

Yes, the diagnosis and evaluations are difficult times that don't go away. They're confusing and painful. But most of us try not to think about it. I know some people who have learned how to beat the tests. And there are some who have actually found something positive about living with memory loss. Can you imagine that?

John

To Whom I May Concern

Many of the projects that I describe in this section endeavor to bring people fully into the moment. The challenge these programs face is to find ways to capture the power of the moment so they can share it with others who weren't there. With memory loss and dementia, repeating or even expressing one's thoughts or actions becomes the quintessential challenge. Family and caregivers might complain about the opposite— that people with dementia repeat themselves constantly. But the meaningful moments of exchange and self-expression can seem to evaporate in a heartbeat. Or by the time a person with memory loss pulls together thoughts and the courage to share them, the conversation has already moved so far downstream he or she doesn't bother to enter it.

To Whom I May Concern is both a play and a technique for creating and presenting a play based on the words of people with early memory loss. It is also *acted* by people with early memory loss. In essence, the play is a mechanism that allows people with memory loss to recreate moments in which they eloquently express a full range of emotions and ideas: humor, anger, longing, fear, frustration, love, and hope. And it does this through the power of the word, the very thing that so often betrays people with memory loss. The play also gives people with early memory loss a chance to stop the rapid current for a moment, to slow down the speed of communication long enough to be heard.

To Whom I May Concern emerged out of a dissertation by Maureen Matthews, who graduated from New York University with a PhD in nursing in 2005. Matthews ran support groups for people in early stages of memory loss in the New York City area, and she interviewed the participants to better understand their experiences. Hoping to bring her data to life and to encourage readers to empathize with her subjects, Matthews created a play out of the interviews.

Soon after earning her doctorate, Matthews suggested that the New York City chapter of the Alzheimer's Association include a play in its Early Stage Forum, a remarkable conference geared specifically toward people with memory loss. The chapter was one the first in the country to recognize the unique needs of people in the early stages of memory loss, who are often deeply entrenched in "normal" lives—filled with work, friends, family, dreams of the future, and the expectation and ambition to achieve them. In 2006, the New York City chapter held its eighth Early Stage Forum. At other dementia care conferences, professional caregivers gather to talk about best practices in providing care. At this conference, people with memory loss gather to talk about things like how to keep their jobs as long as possible. When Matthews suggested the play idea to the members of the conference planning committee, they jumped on it. "The planning committee loved the idea," said Jed Levine, chapter vice president. "It was interesting, innovative, entertaining, and educational."

The chapter hired Matthews to create a new script based on interviews with volunteers from two Manhattan support groups and hired New York–based theater artist Lauren Volkmer to direct it. Matthews visited the groups and found 10 people who wanted to play. They met with Matthews and Volkmer at the Alzheimer's Association offices just south of Grand Central Station once a week for 4 weeks. The group shared their experiences with early memory loss, and Matthews edited their accounts into letter form.

In May 2006, the auditorium at the CUNY Graduate Center in Manhattan was filled with some 300 people gathered for the conference. The actors included one person with performing experience, but otherwise, they were all newcomers to projecting their voices and conquering stage fright. And, of course, they all had memory loss. They had rehearsed for weeks. But Matthews and Volkmer weren't sure what would happen.

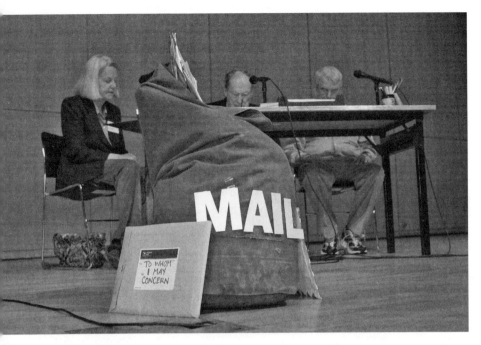

To Whom I May Concern, performed at the Early Stage Forum of the Alzheimer's Association, New York City chapter, in May 2006. Photo by Ronald L. Glassman.

The play opens with John, the narrator, sitting at a desk writing a letter. An oversized and overflowing mailbag sits next to him. John introduces the "letters" framework for the play as he reads:

To whom *I* may concern:

I know, you think I've made a mistake. You think I meant to write "To Whom *It* May Concern." But don't worry. It's not a mistake. This is not just any letter to some unknown person or persons, a form letter that complains or advises.

No, this letter is not about an "It" that may concern you, but of an "I," that is, me. I am writing to you today to let you know what it is like to be *me* these days.

John was the only actor with professional performing experience, having done regional theater and even some Broadway. "When John came on," said Volkmer, "he was sparkling. He was in the moment, in his element." Then about halfway through the play, he lost his place in the script. "We could see it," said Volkmer, "he was flipping through the script. But he was too far away for others to help him. He was starting to panic. He knew it was his turn, but he had no idea what he was supposed to do." Matthews said, "It was awkward. The audience didn't know if it was part of the play or not. You could feel the tension in the room." Then a fellow performer walked over and pointed out his place in the script. John stood up, looked out at the audience, and said. "Sorry about that. I have Alzheimer's." The tension melted. Laughter and applause swelled.

In the first section of the play, the letters focus on diagnosis. Margaret thoughtfully compels her doctor to have a little more understanding.

Dear Doctor:

Today was terrifying. I felt so alone. I couldn't believe those words were coming out of your mouth: "Margaret, you have probable Alzheimer's disease and you have to take all this medicine and we just have to see what happens with it. And then come back in 6 months."

I wish you could have told me more about what to expect. What's going to happen to me? What should I do about it?

It was like my whole world fell apart. I was in a daze. After I left your office I just stood outside the hospital, wondering what my next move should be.

I'm enclosing the phone number of Alzheimer's chapter. When I asked you for it, you couldn't find it. It might be a good thing to hang on to because it might be the only thing someone like me can hang on to.

See you in 6 months.

Margaret

Richard, on the other hand, cuts current diagnostic practices to the quick:

Dear Doctor,

I just spent $5,000 to learn what I knew when I came into your office in the first place: I have probable Alzheimer's disease. Do you think I got my money's worth?

Sincerely,

Your *probable* patient,

Richard

Other letters are directed to God (give me strength), Barnes and Noble (you have books for caregivers, but where are the books for people with memory loss?), the assessment team (be honest with me), and colleagues. Margaret writes to the head of a professional organization in her field:

> When I received word today that I was no longer wanted, I was devastated. Of course, you didn't use those words. You said that membership was limited and you had already taken in your quota of new members for the year. But I saw one of your members' reaction when I shared with her that I had been diagnosed with Alzheimer's disease. How naïve I was that she would not be prejudiced and that she would not communicate this to the membership committee.
>
> I hope you will educate yourselves about the impact of Alzheimer's disease, especially for those in the early stages. I am still very much a part of the world and I'm not contagious.

The overall tone of the letters is a deft balance of humor, anger, anxiety, and hope. Says one man, "Sometimes I like to picture the doctors as Groucho Marx when he played Dr. Hugo Z. Hackenbush, MD, PhD, RFD, MD, PDQ, BYOB." But overall, the effect is of a shaken bottle of soda being uncapped. Effervescent, sweet, unpredictable, and a bit explosive.

To Whom I May Concern had an enormous impact on its audience. The way the work was crafted, the integrity of the environment that Matthews and Volkmer created, has, in Jed Levine's opinion, enormous potential to change attitudes of a wide range of people, including family members, people with memory loss, doctors, even members of the pharmaceutical industry. One story Levine told me was emblematic of the response to the play. A gentleman with memory loss attended the conference with his wife. After the play, he told a staff member of the Alzheimer's Association that the play showed him for the first time people with memory loss he didn't dismiss as crazy or dysfunctional. For the first time, he found people he could relate to. He and his wife have both since joined several groups at the association. Levine also told of a neurologist who responded to the play by saying, "Every doctor who diagnoses dementia should see this."

The second production of *To Whom I May Concern*, which took place in 2007, was brought about by a grant from the Society for the Arts in Healthcare in collaboration with Artists for Alzheimer's, a program that coordinates and nurtures artists who volunteer in dementia care settings, particularly in the New York City area. Matthews and Volkmer worked with an early memory loss support group in Little Neck (Queens/Long Island), this time producing the play themselves at a community center and then at the Long Island Alzheimer's Foundation.

The second version of *To Whom I May Concern* follows the same basic format as the first, but the individual letters capture the unique voices of the Queens participants. May writes to a museum docent, thanking her for taking her group's request not to speak so slowly to them so well: "You were very gracious when someone in our group spoke up and assured you that you could speak to us like any other group of adults. You actually seemed relieved. *We* certainly were."

Adele reads a letter to her husband, who was in the audience.

> I don't mean to sound ungrateful or rude, but I have to tell you that you're being overly helpful. Ever since the doctor said I might have Alzheimer's disease, you have been watching over me like a hawk. Now I'm not saying that I don't like the attention. Actually, it's very nice because you're being so thoughtful. But sometimes it can be infantilizing. I know that's not your intent, but that's how it feels. I know my memory isn't good. I'm forgetting all kinds of things. I start a sentence and I can't remember what I wanted to say. Sometimes you remind me and that can be very helpful. The problem is when you *assume* I'm going to forget.

While Adele was reading the letter, she looked directly at her husband. The content of the letter was difficult, and, according to Volkmer, Adele likely hadn't said the words out loud before. "I felt like we were witnessing something special," Volkmer said. In the postshow discussion, Adele's husband stood up. He thanked her, and the play, for opening his eyes to her feelings.

This moment of exchange between Adele and her husband in particular crystallized Matthews's thoughts about the power of the play. Having immersed herself in readings about theater ethnography and Augusto Boal's *Theater of the Oppressed*, Matthews sees *To Whom I May Concern* as a chance for people who are silenced to speak. "This is an opportunity for people who lose their voice to disease to enter into dialogue with those who accompany them," said Matthews. "The play itself is only a piece of it. A critical piece is the interaction with the audience."

Other letters in the Queens script both mock and sincerely thank

Access-a-ride and testify to the life preserver that is their support group. Anne, the narrator of the Queens script, gets the final word: "I also try to forget. I know that may sound funny . . . forgetting is at the heart of my problem. But I do try to forget about dementia. I don't want it to define me. I'm more than my memory. Let's have some fun."

Like StoryCorps' Memory Loss Initiative (MLI), *To Whom I May Concern* invites us to dam the rushing waters of our lives long enough to allow people with memory loss to collect and share their thoughts with us. Both projects invite us to listen, really listen, and to see just how often we waste our moments and opportunities for deeply connecting to others. And like MLI, *To Whom I May Concern* creates a tangible mechanism for sharing those moments with others—in this case a play.

Matthews and Volkmer dream of being able to create *To Whom I May Concern* plays all over the country. Surveys completed by audience members before and after the two Queens / Long Island performances suggest that the play has an impact on people's attitudes toward memory loss. Matthews is eager to do more interviewing about the impact of the project, and she sees potential in expanding it to people with other disabilities. Volkmer dreams of making a film out of the project so that it can reach larger audiences. A film would reduce some of the performers' anxiety, but it would also drain a little of the power out of the play— power and tension that come from the magic of a live performance, where anything can happen. Even the radical act of listening.

Time*Slips* Creative Storytelling Project

❧ Write this down. This story was made up by the old people at the Catholic Home, who don't just sit here but we think. Everyone has an idea. You should publish this in the *Reader's Digest*. They should publish this in the paper.

Gretchen

"His name is Piggy Wiggy," says a man with a wry grin. He sits in a half circle of 20 chairs filled with participants of Luther Manor Adult Day Center.

"Where should we say this is?" asks a young woman in the middle of the half circle.

The group is looking at a black and white copy of a picture of a polar bear, sprawled on his stomach on the ice, with glasses propped on the top of his head. He appears to be reading a newspaper.

"What is he doing?" asks the young woman. Another woman with smartly cut white hair stands next to her. Quickly and neatly, she captures every word in flawless cursive on the flip chart.

"I would feed him," says a woman. "He would eat some chicken and collard greens."

"Bears don't eat greens," says another storyteller.

"Well, *I* would feed him greens," says the first, laughing.

"I would take him to church," says another woman.

"People would run out," laughs a man.

"Not the preacher—he *has* to stay!"

"Mmmm hmmmm!" say several storytellers.

"That's right," echo others.

The young woman is breaking a sweat as she moves about, trying to follow the energy flying around the room.

This scene takes place in June 2007, in Milwaukee, Wisconsin. Eleven years earlier, I had been the one sweating in the semicircle, juggling a story born of asking open-ended questions about a magical picture to a dozen older men and women whom the world thinks have lost themselves. Then I would look up at the faces of the onlookers—CEOs, nursing home administrators, family members—in the back of the room and see them frozen in that open smile/laugh, their eyes stuck in a squint: "Is this really happening?" their eyes ask. "Do these people *really* have dementia?" Now, I'm one of those people. I've been doing these Time*Slips* storytelling workshops for 10 years. And when the stories get flying, stories full of humor, sorrow, hope, and regret, it still feels like a miracle.

I began Time*Slips* in 1995 when I moved to Milwaukee for the first time. I had been released into the world with a freshly minted PhD in theater studies. My dissertation lauded the ability of theater to transform the lives of older adults. I interviewed and followed countless men and women involved in the "senior theater" movement—the Geritol Frolics from Brainerd, Minnesota, the Grandparents Living Theatre in Columbus, Ohio, the Roots and Branches Theater Company in New York City. These performers had imagined that aging would bring decline, rigidity, and isolation. Instead, they found themselves playing Juliet or Lear. They received professional training and became comedians, dancers, or singers. They learned to shape their memories into monologues. They found a social network to catch them if they fell and praise them when they excelled. Playing a new role (Juliet, Lear, or themselves reborn) radically changed the experience of aging for these performers, their families, and their audiences.

When I moved to Milwaukee in 1995, I had a fellowship that gave me the luxury of a full year to think and write about acting and aging and acting one's age. The question that haunted me was whether the power of performance could transform the lives of older men and women with dementia as it clearly did the lives of those without cognitive disabilities.

By happenstance, a cousin of my father's arranged for me to volunteer at a nursing home. Once a week I made the trek to the edge of town, doubts and fears piling atop each other as my little Corolla rolled me closer to the smells, yells, and alarms that I had come to dread. For 6 weeks I tried. I researched creative dramatics, but the exercises that seemed to work with other groups fell flat with my little group at the nursing home. They seemed shackled—by drugs, by disease, by disinterest. Still, I tried. "Be a tree. Now be a tree in the wind." Nothing.

"Imagine a holiday. What are the smells of Christmas? The sounds?" Nothing. No one talked. No one moved. They watched me, when they were able to hold up their heads, with what could be described only as a blend of pity and apology. We all labored to hear each other through the blaring game shows and the sound of mass playing on transistor radios in the laps of a group of nuns in the corner of the chaotic common room. The alarm, which went off when someone "wandered" past a threshold, seemed permanently triggered. I ached for them. But I couldn't reach a single one of them.

Something happened in the seventh week. I gave up on memory, of trying to trigger thoughts of the past. Instead, I tore a picture of the Marlboro Man from a magazine and dragged along with me a big pad of newsprint paper and a box of markers. I gathered the group, and we sat down around our usual table in the common room. I blocked out the overpowering sounds and smells, keeping my concentration and remaining calm.

"Forget about remembering," I said. "Let's make it up." "What should we call this guy? You can say anything you want, and I'll write it down. Anything."

"Fred," said one woman, breaking a smile.

"Fred who?" I asked, shocked at the response.

"Fred Astaire."

And so it began. I felt short of breath. I kept asking questions.

"Where does he live?"

"Oklahoma."

And someone sang, "Oklahoma, where the wind comes sweeping down the plain."

"What is Oklahoma like?"

"There are lots of skinny rivers and skinny trees."

"What does he eat?"

"Fish. Two for breakfast, two for lunch, two for dinner. He's sick of fish."

The story went on for 45 minutes. By the end, we knew that Fred Astaire was married to Gina Autry. They didn't have kids, because they didn't have time. They did have three dogs, and they tended black and white cows that said, "Hi, Pat." They performed in rodeos—she did the barrel riding and he roped calves. She was better than he was. They had a big Christmas dinner. They served goose on a white tablecloth.

At the end of the 45 minutes, we were all in a kind of shock. I looked around our little table and noticed that, for the first time in 7 weeks, a couple of staff members had wandered over to see what the ruckus was about. There had been a double transformation. Becoming storytellers had transformed the residents *and* the staff.

Of course, every week from then on I did the same thing, trying to see if the magic could happen again.

Twelve weeks later, we had told more than a dozen stories. I still had to suppress the gag reflex each time I walked through the door of the nursing home. The alarm still shattered our concentration. But we also laughed, sang, and told stories together. We'd found a way to reach each other. My weekly trip in the Toyota was now a blend of apprehension and eager anticipation.

It is April 2007. The polar bear sprawled out on the ice is "reading the stock report," said June. Five students from my storytelling class in the Theatre Department at the University of Wisconsin–Milwaukee are asking the questions.

"What happens next?"

"He falls through the ice."

"Oh! And then what?"

This bear had already survived two or three other falls as he made his way toward a sexy black bear just beyond his ice floe. "He dies," says June, one of the students' favorite storytellers. She peers at them through her enormous glasses with one dark lens and one empty lens, dramatically revealing a brilliant blue eye. The students seem heartbroken. Beulah, another storyteller, senses the students' shock, and counters, "He doesn't die. You have to have something to live for." June closes her eyes and pauses for a moment. Then she starts to sing. "Que sera sera, whatever will be, will be." The students and storytellers join in—the hard reality of death and loss softened by the joining of voices.

It is winter 1999. A woman wearing some sort of Victorian costume is riding an ostrich. The storytellers, gathered in the basement of a synagogue in midtown Manhattan, name her "Holding On—because she's really just *holding on*." She is a cancan dancer, comfortable with herself, contemplating the next move in her career. "She never had children," says Betty, "and she thinks she might have missed something. But she has a complex sense of happiness."

It is fall 2003. After a raucous storytelling session at Luther Manor, we are all a little giddy from the humor and energy that lingers in the room. No one gets up. We don't want it to end. One of the storytellers leans forward and calls the group to attention. "Hey!" she says, "we're a group here! And we're really good!"

We're in Brooklyn in 1999. In an old Robert Doisneau photograph, a woman dressed in a heavy winter coat sits reclined on a Paris park bench. The painter standing in front of her has captured the essence of her reclining figure but drawn her as an abstract nude. The women storytellers at the Park Slope Geriatric Day Center begin to twitter. "What should we call the woman?" asks one of the New York University students leading the group. "Mildred!" "Betty!" "Ida!" The three women shout out their own names—suddenly and playfully transforming themselves into the young, curvaceous woman on the Parisian bridge.

From my weekly journey in my Corolla in 1995 to today, Time*Slips* has grown quite a bit. In 1998, the Brookdale Foundation and the Helen Bader Foundation supported a 2-year evaluation of the project, in which we taught others to do it and interviewed staff, families, and student facilitators about if and how it worked. We also shared the stories with public audiences and asked them if it changed their attitudes about memory loss and dementia. I wrote and staged three different plays based on the stories. The first, staged in Oshkosh, Wisconsin, in 1997, was based on those original stories gathered in the Milwaukee nursing home. Fred Astaire the cowboy was played by a man in his 70s and an 8-year-old boy simultaneously. In 2000, we staged a play based on stories from the Milwaukee storytelling groups, and in 2001, we staged one in New York based on stories that emerged there.

The plays were powerful experiences. Each one featured characters and storylines created by people with dementia. They seemed to conjure the storytellers themselves, and each performance became a kind of incantation. This effect wasn't as strong in the Oshkosh production, likely because the stories had come from Milwaukee, and there were no family members at the production. But for the Milwaukee production in 2000, we invited the staff, storytellers, and their families to the professional theater production. One of the stories featured Ethel Rebecca, an octogenarian pilot flying to Seattle with Dizzy Gillespie in the backseat of her antique plane. A storyteller named Mary had given Ethel Rebecca a song to sing with Dizzy, an Italian-American song, the lyrics of which took me several months to track down. In the Milwaukee production, Ethel was played by Adekola Adedapo, a local jazz singer. In the opening moments of the show, Adedapo, wearing a bomber jacket, leather

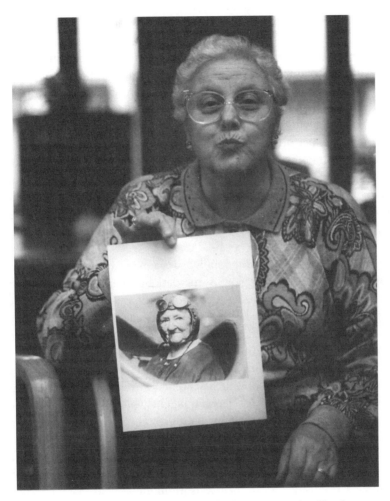

Mary tells a story about a pilot named Ethel Rebecca who flies because it makes her feel free. Photo by Dick Blau.

helmet, goggles, and a white flowing scarf, ran at full speed up a ramp, a white handheld fan acting as her propeller, and landed in the middle of the audience, where she belted out "Cera Luna Mezza Mara Mamma Mia Mi Mari Dari!" On opening night, I panicked when I saw that Mary's husband was sitting in front of the ramp. Adekola would shortly be singing, at full lung capacity, right into his face. Lights were going down, there wasn't time to let him know, to offer to let him move to another seat. After the show, I approached him sheepishly. "What did you think of the show?" "Mary was right there with me," he said. "Is it okay if I come again?" He sat in the same seat for two other performances.

All three plays aimed to capture the breathless surprise of creativity emerging from someone the world has written off. The Oshkosh and Milwaukee plays dove into the world of the characters created by the storytellers, relying on the play program and the "talk back" session that followed the performance to provide context. In the opening scene in the Oshkosh performance, the 8-year-old boy playing cowboy Fred Astaire crawled out of the top drawer of a highboy dresser, pulling a suitcase behind him. He opened the suitcase, set it down, sat in it, pulled out his fishing pole, and began to fish, singing "One, two, three, four, five, once I caught a fish alive. Six, seven, eight, nine, ten, then I threw it back again."

In the Milwaukee production in 2000, a man wearing a bathing suit, flippers, and goggles with glow-in-the-dark lights around the lenses and fish in his hair walked on stage through one of a series of doors, opened a suitcase on the stage, and, literally, dove in. The director of both plays, Gülgün Kayim, created stage images that suggested that there were no boundaries to the world of the imagination.

The imagination didn't go unchallenged in the plays, however. In the Milwaukee production, the first scene featured each character playing a bit of the storyline. An elephant juggles while telling his story, fearing that he's repeating himself. Two nuns recount the tale of their fishing prowess. A artist paints while his model fights boredom. A pilot races upward into the "sky," on her way to teach her granddaughter to fly. And then the second scene repeats the first, almost exactly. Just as the audience begins to shift in their seats, thinking—"Was that a mistake?" "Didn't we just see that?" "How long will this repetition go on?"—the scene breaks, and small changes take place. Objects that are heavily identified with each character begin to circulate. The swimmer's flippers, for example, migrate to one of the nuns. During the third scene, the objects are in a free-for-all. The elephant wears the artist's easel. The nuns play with the swimmer's beach ball. But somehow, their stories progress. In the final scene, there are almost no words left. Simple movements tell the stories we've heard repeatedly and come to know. The characters help complete each other's stories by filling in a word or movement here, an object there.

Like the experience of dementia itself, these characters and their stories become distilled. Ideally, the audience, by learning the characters' unique languages, can understand them even when they are beyond words.

After each performance in Milwaukee and New York, we held "talk backs" as a way for people to process what they'd seen. One evening, two women, who were sitting next to each other, had powerful and opposite responses to the Milwaukee play production. The first woman answered the facilitator's call for reactions to the play. "When that scene started to repeat, I almost left," she said, her voice shaking. "I couldn't stand the repetition. There is *no* sense to Alzheimer's. *None*." Her friend countered, in gentle tones: "I felt the opposite. When the scene started to repeat, I thought—oh no. But then I started to see things. Even when they were just making movements, it made sense to me. I felt I knew them."

I worried for their friendship, but I was thankful for their deeply felt responses. They seemed to capture the range of emotions surrounding dementia. Anger and hopelessness, on the one hand. Openness to mystery and hope in human connection, on the other.

In the New York production in 2001, director Christopher Bayes, nationally known for his work in clowning, turned in a different direction. We put the storytelling process on stage to show people from whence the fanciful characters and storylines came. Bayes's production, with its magical, luminescent folding and unfolding set by David Korins and delicate live music (accordion and violin), grounded the audience before encouraging them to fly away into the world of the imagination. Characters featured Holding On, the Parisian cancan dancer; Thomas Rex and Godfrey (God for short), a cowboy and his singing horse; Bookman, who is trying to make sense of all the books in the world by "orchestrating an orchestra in his mind"; and a swimmer (Marianne) trying to break a record in the Hudson River. The characters shared their tales, but something kept them from completing their stories. Gradually, they filled in each other's gaps. Marianne donned Holding On's tutu and did the cancan. "God" played both parts when Thomas Rex began to lose his words. And in the final moments, all the characters picked up books fastened onto the end of long sticks and moved them together, in unison, like a flock of birds, to finally, finally, fulfill Bookman's dream—to make sense of them.

With hindsight, I can see that the message of all three plays echoes

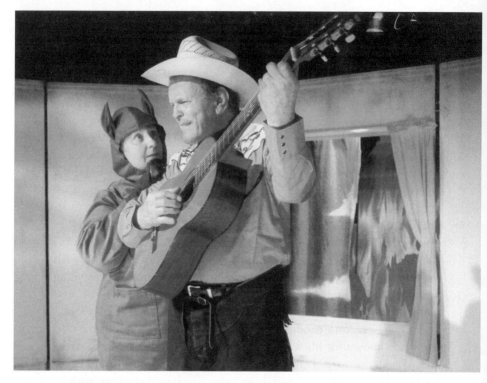

Godfrey (Jodie Lynn McClintock) and Thomas Rex (Michael Shelle) in
the New York TimeSlips play, 2001. Photo by Tim Atkinson.

the power of the group storytelling process itself. We all help each other
to complete the stories of our lives. None of us, with or without memory loss, can complete a story alone.

It's June 2007. There are three storytelling sessions happening simultaneously at the Luther Manor Adult Day Center in Milwaukee. They are
being facilitated by a blend of experienced Time*Slips* trainers from across
the country (there are now 30 trainers covering 10 different states) and
staff and volunteers from Luther Manor. There is laughter, song, shared
excitement, and energy. I'm just watching in the background, my mouth
half open, looking to the other observers around me for confirmation—
"Is this really happening?" "Do they *really* have dementia?"

People with dementia are sewn into figurative straightjackets by institutions (Luther Manor excepted, thankfully) that tell them they are
diseased, inappropriate, challenging, passive objects in need of care—

"the living dead." And somehow, a black and white picture, a marker, a flip chart, and someone asking them what they think and writing down their answers is enough to break those seams.

I Don't Look Like Him!

This is one tired teddy bear or snow bear. He is not blind, but he is cold. His name is Fritz. Fritz is resting because he is very tired, and a teddy bear wouldn't be playing around anyway. He came from the background. He is trying to get some food. He fell through the ice, which surprised him. He is pooped out from trying to get out of the cold water. It is springtime, but it doesn't make much sense that a bear would be out there. Fritz needs to rest until he decides what to do next. But he's glad to be at this point. He's trying to get help from reading to find out how to save himself. He got this book from a friend from one of the buildings back there. Even though he is very tired, he is going to pick himself up once he gets a little bit of energy. There is a juicy animal right out there. It's a little penguin. Fritz gets all excited, but he's not going to catch him. He falls through another hole in the ice. He dies. Oh, we don't know if he's going to die . . . you don't just let people die. "Que sera sera" (*singing*). He has to fight for the privilege to keep going. Fritz is fighting to live. We want it to end lovely.

12

Songwriting Works

When they see— . . . it makes me cry and I can't talk. I'm going to take this (songbook) home and show it to my children so they can take it to my grandchildren.

B. C., age 86

The day after the first Iraq war broke out, Judith-Kate Friedman returned to the Jewish Home in San Francisco, where she'd been working as a musician. Friedman is a talented singer and songwriter in her own right, but when she works in a community setting, she acts as a musical mirror of sorts—establishing relationship and trust and then reflecting people's thoughts through a combination of words and sound. On that particular day, she was working in a unit that serves people who are at the end of life, most of whom have moved beyond rational language. This unit, normally active with the sounds of bustling staff and residents, was almost silent. "I'd been doing this work for so long, and I'd never heard it so quiet," she said. She wondered if the residents were responding to the war; certainly the staff would have been aware of it. Many would likely have relatives who would be called to serve. She wondered how to be most useful in this anxious setting. So she began to stroll and play a gentle instrumental to soothe the atmosphere. Friedman came up with a melody and continued walking and playing, coming to rest with a woman whose words rarely found an order that people around her could understand. The woman looked eager to engage, so Friedman sat down by her and played, mindful to connect with the others in the room as well. In the middle of their conversation of jumbled words, "she looked at me and said, 'And every life is precious in this world.'" Friedman wove it into the melody she was playing.

"Everyday!" added the woman.

"Everyday!" sang Friedman.

"And it's a very wonderful world!" added the woman.

"And peace will find a way," added Friedman.

For the next hour, Friedman played those four lines and a verse to a unit on a different floor that served people with Alzheimer's disease. She asked the residents what they thought was missing from the song. Someone said, "You have to be thankful every day." The song has become a classic in her repertoire.

At the age of 22, after studying music, poetry, and folklore at Oberlin, Judith-Kate Friedman made her way to the San Francisco area, where she stayed for 22 years. She knew she wanted to be a performing songwriter after college, and in pursuit of this dream, she took a variety of part-time jobs. She accepted an invitation by friends working in a nursing home to try playing music there and found she had a nice rapport with the residents. "I never knew my own grandparents, and I thought it would be nice to have relationships with older people," said Friedman. She was also no stranger to disability. Born with a club foot and subjected to multiple surgeries as a child, Friedman was accustomed to fighting for the recognition of people with disabilities as full citizens.

But in the beginning, Friedman sensed that something was missing in the nursing home work. With hindsight, Friedman described most nursing home musical work as "maintenance entertainment," which she sees as a symptom of overworked staff in an institutional setting with institutional "think." In these scenarios, social programming is distributed like a sprinkler—to cover the largest area and the most people as possible. Friedman describes it this way: "There are wonderful teachers out there doing incredibly engaging things. And there are others who have crafted their interaction to keep people happy. It works for everyone. It seems to include people, but there's not a fresh engagement that happens each time that allows for surprise. It's not set up to draw out the individual intelligence."

Certainly "sing-a-long" activities are enjoyable and can build a sense of community. I find myself deeply moved in moments when voices join together—like around the campfire at our annual summer retreat to the Adirondacks, where 30 friends sing show tunes and Pete Seeger songs (hell to some, heaven to me). But Friedman knew she could, and wanted to, go deeper. And the patchwork of part-time sing-a-long gigs was difficult to sustain (if she was to eat at the same time), so she let it go and turned her full attention to writing and recording her own music. Between 1986 and 1989, she recorded her first album and began touring the United States.

Then Robert Rice, at the time head of a California Arts Council program called ArtWorks, invited her to become one of the program's teaching artists and to try something extraordinary. Rice challenged Friedman not just to entertain the people she was working with but to create a meaningful artistic experience for herself as well. He posed a thought-provoking question to her. "He asked me to . . . dig deep as an artist and figure out what would be the most exciting and cutting edge for myself but could also be mutually beneficial for these wonderful people I didn't even know yet. He asked 'What would you do?'"

The first program Friedman tried with this new challenge in mind was at an adult day center in San Francisco. There was a large dayroom and an incredibly diverse group of seniors speaking multiple languages. Two women in the group had walked with Dr. King in Selma. "I suggested to the group that our first song be about Dr. King." One of the women invited Friedman back to her apartment. That conversation, now almost 20 years ago, was remarkable, she says; the visit was "one of the most amazing [ones] with an elder that I've ever had in my life." Working with the elders, Friedman wove the stories the woman told her into one of the verses in the song tribute to Dr. King:

> We started each day with a vision
> And ended each night with a prayer.
> For if you put the Lord first, you stay true to work,
> And the church of your heart is right here.
>
> Martin Luther King changed our world.
> Some people are still trying to live under the same old lies.
> We can't do that anymore.

Robert Rice's challenge to Friedman evolved into what is now known as Songwriting Works (SWW). Founded in 1988, Friedman's program aims to bring people of all ages together with professional songwriters to create and perform original music and transform the quality of life for young and old alike.

Friedman built the program around several core philosophies about which she is deeply fervent. SWW is intentionally inclusive. Friedman always seats people in a circle so everyone can see and hear each other.

In every interaction, in the circle or beyond it, Friedman projects a belief that every human being has musical, creative, and general intelligence: "They are to be honored and respected for being intelligent
people. That's baseline." Participants in SWW share a common challenge that brings them together on equal footing—that of writing a
song together. There are a couple of additional ground rules. SWW sessions aim to generate fully original material. The students and elders she
works with don't write about cartoon or movie characters. Only twice in
18 years and more than 250 original songs has she encountered a lyric
that was borrowed from an old poem. The participants are making their
own art, expressing their own visions.

Once people have gathered in a circle, Friedman starts out with
simple introductions. She explains who she is and why she's there. Then
the brainstorming begins. Friedman might ask what the group is thinking of or launch a provocative question, and a volunteer, armed with a
marker and an easel, captures their responses on paper. "Then I pick up
the guitar, and we figure out what the music is supposed to sound like,"
Friedman says. "We start jamming." Throughout the process, Friedman
listens intently. She listens for nuances, particular styles, rhythms, ca-
dences, patterns, and the meaning and inflection of their words. She and
the group shape all these elements into a song. In one group, for example, there were a lot of veterans. She began by asking them to "tell me
about your war experience." But no one would talk. It was too hard, too
direct. So Friedman found another way in. She asked, "Tell me, what do
you love about this country?" "And this very dignified black woman
said, 'Well, you can serve your god under your own fig tree here.'"
Friedman found the rhythm of the phrase, and the group set it to a tune.
The phrase became the chorus to their song.

In 2001, Friedman worked with a prolific group of elders at the Jewish Home in San Francisco to create more than 40 songs. That summer,
when she won a Best Practices Award from the Association of Jewish
Aging Services, a national organization for Jewish homes and housing
services in North America, the board of the Jewish Home put enough
money behind the project to fulfill one of Friedman's dreams—to "bring
in an engineer and musicians and record it in the home, live, in the synagogue." San Francisco–based filmmaker Nathan Friedkin began visiting
rehearsals September 3, building his footage into *Specially Wonderful
Affair,* a film that has played the festival circuit. Funding secured, filmmaker in place, engineers hired, elders having narrowed their 40 songs

to 13 and at the ready to record, they were set to record on September 12. The events of September 11 changed everything. Should they go on? As she always does, Friedman asked the group for guidance. The oldest member, Birdie Gintzler, who was then 97 and sharp as a tack, gave the definitive response: "If we stop, the terrorists have won." And so they went on, recording the CD *Island on a Hill* with a group of seniors whose average age was 87.

Rabbi Sheldon Marder has been working with Friedman at the Jewish Home since 2002. Together he and Friedman facilitate the Psalms, Songs, and Stories Program, which uses the biblical poetry of the Psalms to express and explore spiritual beliefs through the creation of original songs. Together they meet with two groups of elders, one with dementia, one without. Marder is quick to point out that he's no musician; rather, his aims for the program relate to his mission in pastoral care. "I know Judith-Kate says that we're songwriters, and the point is to write a good song," he says. "For me, the point is not perfection, but significance. And that's exactly what we're aiming for in our songs. They are meant to have significance. They are meant to have meaning or help discover meaning. The fact that they do it together makes it more doable. When people work in a group and give each other ideas, what's hard work becomes fun and exciting. The relationships are at the heart of it."

Marder also uses the songwriting process to learn as much as he can about people moving deeper into memory loss. "A good deal of my work is really just to learn as much about them as I can," says Marder, "and then I remind them of it later on. I know things about people that later surprises them to hear. 'How do you know that about me?' And I tell them, 'You told me about that when we wrote that song together.'"

What is the impact of SWW? Theresa Allison (MD) has been studying SWW at the Jewish Home in San Francisco for several years as part of her dissertation research. Allison has been studying it not as a medical doctor, but, rather, as an ethnomusicologist, conducting unstructured interviews with the residents. She has found that the music that emerges through SWW is deeply interwoven into the very fabric of the Jewish Home. Music from the residents was used as part of the dedication of the synagogue, a ceremony that was reserved for the most generous donors. Several of the residents' songs have landed in the core repertory of the institution. "Everyone on staff knows *It's Hanukah Tonight*," said Allison.

Friedman is adamant that songs written by the groups she serves belong to the group. "The woman who said, 'You can serve your god under your own fig tree here,' that's her line, and it will remain her line for-ever." She tells a story of how when she tried to train another musician to do the SWW process so more people could experience it, the would-be trainee heard someone utter a line he found inspiring and said, "That's a great line. I'm going to use that." Friedman stopped his ap-prenticeship. Says Friedman, "I've got plenty of songs on my own, I don't need [their songs] to be mine. All my skills, my musical skills, all my teaching skills, all my humanities skills go toward assisting people to find and explore and express their inner musicality, their wisdom, and whatever legacy they want to leave and [to] have fun in the process." The issue of ownership becomes especially heated when songs begin building in number and Friedman shares them with the public. When SWW uses the professionally recorded, original music to foster connec-tions between an aging community and the world at large, who profits from the CD sales? All proceeds go back into SWW.

In 2006, Friedman moved her home base to Port Townsend, Wash-ington. After 18 years, 40 different program sites, 250 songs, several CDs, and a documentary film, Friedman started the process of training oth-ers to carry SWW forward. Winning a 2007 MindAlert Award from the MetLife Foundation and the American Society on Aging has helped raise awareness of the program. For now, all the songwriters she has worked with have come out of classroom settings. But that is starting to change with the growth of organizations like the National Center for Creative Aging, based in Washington, D.C., and the Society for the Arts in Health Care, which also addresses aging as part of its mission. "Older arts is not known in the world, at least at this point in time, quite like the genre of children's music." "But," insists Friedman, "this *is* a genre."

She thinks it does take a special personality to be a SWW facilitator. "It takes a lot of patience to be willing to be still within one's self enough to hear the voices of people with dementia. I don't think it's superhuman patience; I think it's an extremely natural thing to do."

Peace Will Find a Way

Every life is precious in this world.
Every day—every day
In this very wonderful world peace will find a way.
   Be thankful—be thankful,
   Thankful every day.

Be thankful—be thankful,
Peace will find a way.
Every day is precious in this life.
Every day—every day
In this very wonderful life love will find a way.
Be thankful—be thankful,
Thankful every day.
Be thankful—be thankful,
Love will find a way.
Be thankful, be thankful—thankful every day.
Be thankful, be thankful—peace will find a way.
Peace will surely find a way.

13

Dance
"Respect" and "Sea of Heartbreak"

❧ At first, I approached this project as I would have any other, but after weeks of seeing each individual eye to eye in our greeting or our closing, I began to really relate to each person as an individual, letting go of my lesson plan for the day, letting go of who was responding and who wasn't. Instead of being the teacher, the leader, I was just part of the group.

Amy Brinkman Sustache

Katie Williams can barely catch her breath. "And Blanche," says Katie, "she's deaf. She can't hear a thing. But she feels the music. She sits right next to me and she watches my movements. She just loves this. She's never missed a show." Then Katie tells me of Robert, about how he is so cautious but just lights up when they dance. And then there's the married couple—the wife who loved the dance program and the husband who sat in a recliner and watched, making snide comments under his breath. Then one day, he quietly asked Katie if he could join the group. And she told me of Ida. And Mary. I couldn't write it all down fast enough. When we got out the scrapbook of the Good Steppers, the Luther Manor dance group, Katie thought of more stories. "Oh! There are our canes! We are so proud of our canes." I'd heard about the canes and hats several times before. They special-ordered them from the Internet.

Katie Williams and Anna Liza Malone are person-centered care specialists at Luther Manor Adult Day Center in Milwaukee, Wisconsin. In other facilities, they would be called "nursing assistants." But at Luther Manor, the concept of befriending participants is built into job descriptions and titles. The ArtCare artist-in-residence program is the epitome of that idea. In 2001, as part of the ArtCare program, a professional choreographer from DanceWorks, a Milwaukee-based nonprofit, was artist in residence at Luther Manor for 15 weeks. It was a mutual exchange.

Dancer and choreographer Amy Brinkman Sustache gave Katie and Anna Liza confidence in their abilities to dance and lead others to do the same. Katie and Anna Liza taught Amy how to work with people with dementia. The weekly dance workshops culminated in a public performance in May 2002. More than 100 people filled the Luther Manor Faith and Education Building. Family members, friends, staff, volunteers, and members of the press sat in neat rows facing the stage. I stood in the back of the room wondering, how will they do this? A rehearsed dance performance? In front of an audience of over 100 people? Many of whom are longing to see their parent or spouse or neighbor as he or she *used to be* not as he or she is?

The performance was stunning. The day center participants filed on stage, some on their own, some assisted by helpers or walkers. Anna Liza and Katie sat among them. Amy, the choreographer, was positioned like a conductor, downstage with her back to the audience. The dancers would follow her movements if they lost their place. But most of the dancers had no trouble remembering the movements, because they had choreographed the dance themselves. The movements were simple, elegant, and sometimes funny. In one, the participants danced with colorful scarves to "Don't Worry, Be Happy." In another, they each said their name and performed a movement to accompany it. I remember low, sweeping movements and jaunty, choppy motions—the self transformed into physical expression.

Dawn Adler, who manages the ArtCare program at Luther Manor, said the key to the success of the Good Steppers program is having the participants generate all the content, from music to props to movements. At first, it seemed, the choreographer wanted to do what she does best—choreograph. But, said Adler, "once she got over that, that's when things really started to happen."

Katie and Anna Liza have been running the Good Steppers since the group's first public performance in 2002. "We ask them what kind of music they want. Everything comes from them," said Anna Liza. Over the years, the group has chosen everything from show tunes to country western songs. One woman loves Elvis, so they've done "All Shook Up." One year they did an international theme. Anna Liza taught them about the culture in her native Philippines and brought in songs that in the United States would be called country western. "We did movements about the culture and the feeling of the music," she said. "We made movements like playing the guitar and women picking vegetables and

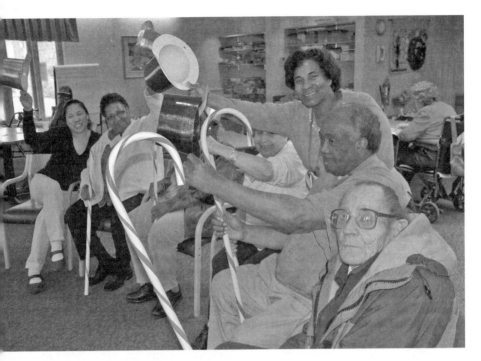

The Good Steppers of Luther Manor. Photo by Anne Basting.

washing rice." The Good Steppers have done everything from Johnny Cash's "Sea of Heartbreak" to Motown with "My Guy." But the favorites are clearly the songs that call for the hats and canes. "We just love our hats," says Katie.

The dancers also pick the movements, props, and costumes. It's a democratic process that demands thinking like a team. "We vote on everything," explains Anna Liza. If someone suggests a movement, they put it up for a vote. For the line "Nothing you can say could tear me away from my guy" in "My Guy," they all tore a piece of construction paper. For "All Shook Up," they put a few kernels of popcorn in plastic water bottles and—shook them up. For "Sea of Heartbreak," they all found white shirts, string ties, and cowboy hats. They found a disco ball for "Saturday Night Fever." The canes and hats come out for "New York, New York," "A Chorus Line," and any other excuse they can find.

Anna Liza and Katie work with the dancers on one song for a couple weeks, then they'll move on to another. When they have finished five songs, the group will rehearse and review and head toward a show. "Some people forget," says Anna Liza, "but that's why Katie and I are there, to remind them and to lead them. We also make a copy of the movement list and put it on the floor in front of each person."

Katie breathlessly tells of how the dancers take to the program. "Della is a loner," she explains. "She does crosswords all day, with the paper right up to her face so she can see it. But when we put on the music, she's the first one there. It's just so much fun to see their eyes light up when we turn on the music."

Several of the projects that I profile in this book encourage people with memory loss to step into the world of imagination as a way to re-connect words to meaning. For many people with memory loss, words are their betrayers. Words slip out of order and relation. They take their sweet time in coming to the lips, or they don't come at all. Sometimes, it doesn't seem worth the risk to wait for them. Time*Slips,* Songwriting Works, Duplex Planet, and StoryCorps, all featured in these chapters, pro-vide ways to enable people with memory loss to express meaning through spoken language. Dance programs, on the other hand, give the body back to people with memory loss. Western culture worships the youth-ful body. It makes the perfect commodity for a capitalist country—an object that gets further from us with each passing moment. Knee re-placements and bypass surgeries are one thing. But we feverishly seek to erase the markings of age that have nothing to do with health and every-thing to do with appearance and social status. Now that "self-esteem" has found a permanent place in the health vernacular, we can rational-ize Botox and plastic surgery as "good" for our health. Dance programs like the Good Steppers provide a way for us to reclaim the aging body, which can be a source of stigma and of physical and emotional pain, as a means of self-expression and a purveyor of pleasure.

Maria Genné, who runs the Kairos Dance Theatre, in Minneapolis, tells a story of a woman with dementia who came to her dance work-shop at a St. Paul adult day center:

> She was very nervous, holding her purse very tightly. She would just sit there and not move or talk, just clutching her purse. I grabbed some Aretha—"Respect" can usually get anybody to dance. And the next thing I knew, there she was, no purse, dancing in the center of the group. And I jumped in to dance with her. And there was joy in the whole group[,] . . . celebrating her being part of us and feeling safe enough to let go of the chair and go into the middle.

Genné has been teaching dance for over 40 years. She began to focus on working with people with memory loss in 2001 after Liz Lerman's Dance Exchange visited Minneapolis as part of that company's Hallelujah project. Genné volunteered to be a liaison for the mammoth Dance Exchange endeavor, in which local communities turned stories into movement based on the question "What are you in praise of?" Genné was placed at the Southwest Senior Center in Minneapolis, a program, coincidentally, Genné's mother had recently begun to visit. Today, Genné's company has several regular sites (adult day programs) it works with each year. There has been compelling research done about the ability of dance and music therapy to reach people with dementia. But Genné and certainly Katie and Anna Liza are coming at the matter from a different perspective. "I'm coming from the artistic process model." says Genné, "It's not about starting with diagnosis. I don't want to know the details. The artist comes in to complement the medical model. We work with chaos and find beauty within it. Art is an expression of the inner person that isn't always described in the medical model."

Liz Lerman puts it in a similar way. She sees the arts as a wide spectrum. On one end, there are therapists dealing with things that only they are trained and able to do. On the other end is an elite, artistic, cultural practice (like opera or ballet) that is pretty removed from everyday people. Says Lerman: "If you remove judgment about the spectrum, you can see this incredibly busy highway between the two ends." The point of entry for her own work is a contract she figuratively signs with participants "that's about 'let's make art,' rather than 'let's make you feel better.'" Of course, there is a lot of overlap in these approaches. But there are not a lot of elite-level artists who can work with such an open-ended process. And, as Lerman suggests, there are also some therapists who don't really want people to be in control of their bodies.

Lerman's company now works with a wide range of community groups, but the Dance Exchange emerged in 1976 out of an ongoing series of workshops at the Roosevelt Hotel for Senior Citizens. Lerman sees all the company's methods for working in community as stemming from those initial years at the Roosevelt, where developmentally disabled people, people with dementia, the poor, and the frail were all lumped together. According to Lerman, in those early days one of the Dance Exchange company members was completely at ease diving deep into the present moment to be with people with memory loss to foster "present time" activities: "That's when I began to muse about memory. Society wants to tell people to live in their memories. Why? They couldn't have new ones? It was shocking to me. Confronting the Alzheimer's situation (and this was before anyone knew what it was) made us question what we were doing. It is fine to ask about 'a time in your life when.' But you can also create it in the moment."

Lerman likes to do what she calls "subtracting meaning" to pull people into the present and get them to think of common things in uncommon ways. A "present time" activity for example, might be to ask people to bring in a family photograph. But instead of telling a story about the people in it, Lerman will guide the dancers through a discussion of the lines, shadows, and shapes they see. "You might get stories of the past," says Lerman, "or you might get art."

I Am a Dancer was the title of the performance at the Luther Manor Faith and Education Building in May 2002 when 18 Luther Manor day center dancers sat on stage, fanned out in a semicircle, and reclaimed their right to find joy in their bodies. *I Am the Running Girl.* That was the title of a book my father gave me when I was 14. It is a kid's book that tells the story of a young girl who learns the power of physical strength, rhythmic movement, and the hypnotic sound of one's own measured breath. That's what I remember, at least. I can see it sitting on the modern, white wall unit in the living room of my parent's old house, but I haven't actually seen it in probably 25 years. *I Am the Running Girl.* When I run my 3-mile route that starts and ends at my front door, I imagine—see and feel—all of my 3-mile routes from the last 30 years. Up Mount Tabor in Portland; around Lake Harriet in Minneapolis; through Prospect Park in Brooklyn. I know there will be a day when my knees will tell a different story. And perhaps, if I'm lucky enough to find a Katie, Anna Liza, Maria, or one of the many people inspired by Liz Lerman, I'll be able to see and feel those places again with a few movements of the arms and hips to a rousing chorus of "Respect."

14

The Visual Arts

✨ It's like he's trying to tell a story with words that don't exist.

Ruben Rosen

In the Metropolitan Museum of Art in New York City is a giant painting by Jackson Pollock. It takes up most of a wall. Its frantic, stringy glops of gray, white, and black paint vibrate across every inch of the enormous canvas. When I first met the man who is now my husband, we spent an afternoon in the Met. He pulled me zigzagging through gallery after gallery to see his favorites. Kandinsky's *Garden of Love,* Bruegel's *Harvesters,* and, of course, Pollock's *Autumn Rhythm, Number 30.* But Brad didn't just *look* at the Pollock. He liked to sit on the bench in front of the painting, and tip backward, lying down to look at the painting upside down. I am more cautious by nature. I looked at the guards first. They seemed okay with this unorthodox viewing method, so I gave it a try. Somehow the painting made perfect sense this way. It was the rest of the world that was upside down. Pollock's *Autumn Rhythm* was in perfect harmony.

When I first looked at the Pollock upside down with Brad, I was just embarking on my journey into understanding the world of dementia. With hindsight, now I wonder, what about those who feel like the world is upside down 24/7? Might Pollock's paintings offer them a similar sense of solace as it offered me? Might this be a place where we could reach each other?

In 2006, Francesca Rosenberg attended a conference hosted by the Council of Senior Centers and Services of New York City. As the director of education at New York's Museum of Modern Art (MoMA), Rosenberg had already been offering programs for seniors and wanted to learn more about this segment of her audience. At the conference, she met Sean Caufield, director of community relations at Hearthstone Alzheimer's Care, who challenged her to think about the growing numbers of older adults with cognitive challenges and their care partners. How was MoMA planning to serve them?

Inspired by Caufield's question, and by the program Artists for Alzheimer's (ARTZ), which Hearthstone had pioneered, Rosenberg called on some local resources to help her shape a program for people with dementia. In addition to Caufield and John Zeisel, ARTZ founder, staff of the New York City chapter of the Alzheimer's Association and specialists from Mt. Sinai Medical Center helped Rosenberg create a training program for museum educators that addressed communication issues, the basics of dementia, and some of the challenges facing caregivers. MoMA educators took prints out into the field to practice at adult day programs. They discovered that some of the classics from their collection, particularly the more representational art, were ideal for igniting conversations full of feeling and poetic expression. Andrew Wyeth's *Christina's World* and Pablo Picasso's *Girl before a Mirror* were instant hits. The test run also revealed that once groups warmed up with Wyeth or Picasso, they could easily move to something less representational— something like Piet Mondrian's *Broadway Boogie Woogie* or Jackson Pollock's *One. One* is remarkably like *Autumn Rhythm Number 30*—so much so that when I sat down to write this chapter, I strained to remember if my date with Brad was at MoMA or the Met. I could picture us wandering the halls of both museums.

When MoMA was still in its temporary home in Queens (while the home campus was being renovated), Rosenberg had some local groups of people with dementia come to the museum for a trial run of the program. When the New York City–based Samuels Foundation funded the program, Meet Me at MoMA was born. In January 2006, on a Tuesday when the museum was closed to the public, MoMA held the first official tour for people with dementia and their care partners. Rosenberg originally thought that the program would run every other month. But the demand became so great that by 2007, MoMA was offering Meet Me at MoMA every month.

On a Tuesday in September 2007, 90 people showed up for the program, which runs from 2:30 to 4:00 in the afternoon. MoMA educators create small groups of no more than 15 people and take each group on a tour of a specific gallery. The power of the program is that it creates a common ground: there are no wrong answers about *Broadway Boogie Woogie;* there are only thought-provoking, emotional responses. The program also honors people with dementia by opening the resources of this magnificent museum to them. A special daylong seminar on the Meet Me at MoMA program in March 2008 featured a panel discussion of participants who eloquently and emotionally described the power of feeling welcomed and honored at a time of life that can be dominated by loss and grief. One woman, whose husband had dementia, said she and her brother would vie for the chance to accompany him to "his" museum for the day. The son of a woman with dementia said his mother treasured the visits and counted down the days until they could visit the museum again. He even scanned postcards from the museum collection into his mother's computer and left the slide show on for her during the day to bring a bit of the museum home to her. Clearly, the program offered participants the chance to suspend or bracket the disease that so dominated their days to create moments of shared joy, learning, and deep engagement.

Making Art

Originally, MoMA staff had hoped to include workshops in which participants could make their own art as well, but logistics made this nearly impossible. Physically moving through the galleries and allowing enough time for in-depth discussion with 15 people didn't leave time to get participants to the workshop spaces. With such a world-class collection ready and waiting for them alone, some participants were invested mainly in the looking, not in the making. But several well-established programs across the country do offer art making for people with dementia, and their results are inspirational.

ArtCare

Luther Manor's adult day program in Milwaukee features an artist in residence each year. In 2006–7, that artist was Michalene (Mollie) Groshek, a lifelong teaching artist who facilitated weekly workshops in which people with dementia worked with mixed media, including ink, fabric, and paint. Mollie fills each art-making moment with choices. Oreda began one of Groshek's art-making sessions by dropping india ink on paper and then turning the paper to allow it to flow in different directions. In the course of doing so, she got some ink on her hands. As she blotted her hands and the artwork with paper towels, she created even more patterns. When it was all dry, she selected collage cutouts, images from magazines, and small pieces of cut tissue paper and layered the work with pastel chalk.

Like all Luther Manor residencies, Groshek's shared the fruits of the participants' labor with the public. Luther Manor sent out formal invitations to press, families, and guests for a reception and a tour of the exhibit housed in their beautiful and newly renovated welcome center. The vibrantly painted fabrics and richly textured collages were professionally mounted, framed, and photographed. I wandered through the exhibit, the sun pouring through windows illuminating the bright fabrics, thinking about how the care with which Mollie presented the artwork models respect for people with cognitive challenges. We weren't just seeing art at this exhibit; we were learning how to see people with dementia.

Artists for Alzheimer's (ARTZ)

Based at Hearthstone Alzheimer's Care, ARTZ has ambitious goals that include both art making and art viewing. Each artist in their sizable stable of volunteers offers a minimum of 1 hour (or one visit) per year to work with people with dementia. When I last visited the Web site, there were 56 artist profiles. Some are professional artists—painters, pianists, sculptors, storytellers, actors, percussionists, and poets—looking for a meaningful way to share their talents. Others are ensconced in careers as care managers, pharmaceutical representatives, or teachers and are looking to work with people with memory loss in ways that their career paths don't permit. ARTZ trains artists in a daylong workshop and then matches them up with a member organization. Each artist can choose to present their craft to the group or to facilitate art making. A poet, for example, might read poetry to a group or work with the group to help them to write their own poems. As an organization, ARTZ is working to expand the use of the arts to empower people with dementia across the globe; it currently has chapters in Germany, Australia, and France and soon will have one in England. In addition to consulting on the formation of the MoMA program, Caufield and founder John Zeisel created an art exhibit called *I'm Still Here* that premiered at the John Kohler Art Center, in Sheboygan, Wisconsin, and appeared in the lobby of Merck. Caufield coordinates the comings and goings of ARTZ volunteer artists and member organizations. Zeisel describes ARTZ's lofty goals this way: "We want every cultural institution *everywhere* to open their doors to people with dementia—they should all be treatment resources. We want to reduce the stigma of the disease, and we want the entire effort to

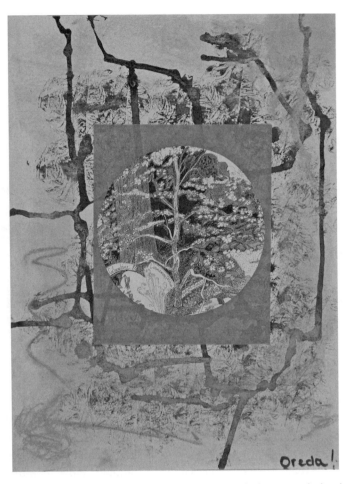

Mixed media collage by Oreda. Her teacher is Michalene Groshek. Photo by Bill Lemke, used with permission of Michalene Groshek.

be self-sustaining." ARTZ supplies training to the staff of organizations that become members about how to work with artists, receive visits from volunteer artists, and gain access to free tickets for cultural events such as the Big Apple Circus, poetry readings, and film screenings.

Arts for the Aging (AFTA)
Like ARTZ, AFTA has assembled a similar range of artists, but AFTA calls them "faculty" and trains and pays them to offer ongoing work-

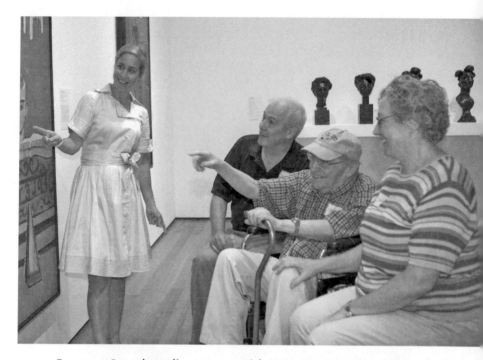

Francesca Rosenberg discusses art with Meet Me at MoMA participants.
Photo by Robin Holland.

shops at partnering adult day programs, senior centers, and not-for-profit
long-term care facilities in the Washington, D.C., area that care for the
underserved. The average tenure of an artist on faculty is 9 years. I spent
the day at their Bethesda offices in 2002. Janine Tursini, then program
director, drove me around to visit a couple programs in action: a quiet
poetry workshop for frail elders; a portrait drawing group at a senior
center; and a raucous sing-a-long at a packed-to-the-gills adult day program. In all three, you could see the hard casings of anxiety and confusion that enveloped some of the participants at the beginning of the session crack and fall away.

Founded by sculptor Lolo Sarnoff in 1988, AFTA was early to recognize the power of fostering self-expression and emotional communication through the arts among people who are left socially isolated. In
2006, Tursini became the executive director, and the program is thriving. "We can't do more than what we're doing for more people," said

Tursini, "and we're busting at the seams with the need." Tursini hopes to develop AFTA's artist training program so that it can meet the needs in the Washington, D.C., area. In 2007, AFTA's programs were featured in the documentary *Do Not Go Gently*, by Melissa Godoy and Eileen Littig, and as the film screens around the country, AFTA is offering workshops on a national basis as well. Tursini is inspired by Sarnoff, who turned 91 in 2007. "She's been active her entire life," said Tursini, "and she continues to be involved. She was the visionary, the founder, and a living embodiment of what it means to always create and always be involved in life."

Elders Share the Arts (ESTA)

Founded by Susan Perlstein in 1979, ESTA began with Perlstein's work in the street theater movement and has evolved to offer a wide array of arts-based programming to underserved elders, including people with memory loss, in the New York City area. ESTA programs blend oral history with creative arts to transform memories into art. The Living History Arts programs it offers include intergenerational workshops (Generating Community), exhibits of artwork by older, self-taught artists (Discoveries), and stories crafted and performed by older adults (Bearing Witness). ESTA partners with senior centers or long-term care facilities and conducts a series of workshops that culminate in a celebration each spring called the Living History Festival. These programs are designed to be flexible, and facilitating artists can adapt them to work with people with a range of disabilities, including dementia.

Incredible teaching artists have been associated with ESTA over the years. I had the privilege of watching Peggy Pettitt facilitate an intergenerational group project in Bushwick, Brooklyn, centered on sharing stories about the importance of voting. I first met founder Susan Perlstein in 1995 when I started coming to New York to study the work being done there with older people in the arts. I remember sitting in her Brooklyn apartment, sipping tea and talking about her early work in the VA hospitals in the Bronx. Keeping ESTA alive and thriving over 30 years and leading the field by founding the National Center for Creative Aging demanded street smarts, philanthropy savvy, and an endless supply of raw energy. I wondered how she did it. Then I looked around. There were countless paintings on the walls and in-process canvases on the floor. "These are yours?" I asked. "Yes," she said. Now I see where she gets her calm.

Memories in the Making (MIM)

Watercolor is the medium of choice for the MIM program, first developed by Selly Jenny of the Orange County chapter of the Alzheimer's Association back in 1986. Since then, Alzheimer's Association chapters across the country (the Colorado, Greater Cincinnati, and Greater Wisconsin chapters, for example) have taken it on, deepening it with their own strengths. La Doris Heinly, who goes by Sam, assumed the mantle of training people to do MIM when Jenny died after a long battle with cancer. Heinly created manuals and a book, *Still Here,* which shows the artwork and guides people through the process of offering themes to the painters, nurturing discussion about memories triggered by those themes, and capturing in watercolor the images inspired by those memories. The MIM program has become a standard feature of many Alzheimer's Association chapters' fundraising efforts, with framed paintings offered at silent or live auctions. Many chapters also create greeting cards and calendars of the artwork.

Whether art-making programs work with clay, watercolor, or fabric, however, almost all boil down to the same basic idea. The visual arts offer a way to communicate beyond words. A person can still tell others how he or she feels about the world through color, shape, and texture when his or her tongue ceases to cooperate.

Talking Art

Viewing and talking about art, as in the MoMA program, offers a similar expressive freedom to making it. Sure there are people who can tell us about the social and historical context that Pollock's work builds on. But at the end of the day, looking at the Pollock, right side up or upside down, what does it make us think and feel? "It's like he's trying to tell a story using words that don't exist," said Meet Me at MoMA participant Rueben Rosen of Picasso's *Girl before a Mirror.* In response to Wyeth's *Christina's World,* Irene Brenton said, "You can't see her face, but looking at her, you get the feeling that she's happy." When asked why, Mrs. Brenton responded, "Because you know she's going to get to the house. I'd like to go into that house, too."

The MoMA program was not the first to take seriously the challenge of making collections accessible to people with dementia and their families. The Bruce Museum of Arts and Science in Greenwich, Connecticut, and the Museum of Fine Arts in Boston expanded their accessibility programs, which most commonly address movement, hearing, and sight impairments, to include people with cognitive challenges. MoMA, however, is determined to share what it learned with museums across the country. With a grant from the MetLife Foundation, the MoMA Alzheimer's Project is creating training manuals and holding workshops to foster partnerships between museums and Alzheimer's Association chapters across the country. MoMA is also partnering with a research institution to evaluate the program—to try to quantify just how seeing and talking about art improves quality of life. The ripple effect of the MoMA Alzheimer's Project is already being felt around the country. Rosenberg's team is making presentations on the project at several conferences across the country. The Metropolitan Museum of Art in New York has launched its own program, as have the Frist and the Brooks museums in Tennessee, the Harwood Museum of Art in Taos, New Mexico, the Virginia Museum of Fine Arts in Richmond, and the Los Angeles County Museum of Art. Clearly, the idea of cultural institutions becoming part of the treatment, as John Zeisel says, is one whose time has come.

The impact and value of the art experience for people with dementia, whether making it or talking about it, depends—pardon the pun—on how you frame it. Wassily Kandinsky, who was a notoriously labored and deliberate artist in the early years of his career, began to draw more loosely and quickly in his later years as he moved through dementia. Arguments about the value of his late work swirl in the pages of art journals. Was he conscious of what he was doing? Was he simply "demented?" Do his late drawings have any value?

The paintings of William Utermohlen also call the framing into question. A professional artist whose figurative paintings appeared in galleries across the United States and Europe, Utermohlen was diagnosed with Alzheimer's disease in 1995 and endeavored to paint his journey through the disease in collaboration with a team of physicians who studied the changes in his perception and artistic skills. An exhibit of his work toured the country in 2006 in commemoration of his life and the hundredth anniversary of the first diagnosis of Alzheimer's in 1906. Nearly every article that profiles the exhibit reads it as a linear portrait of decline. The Associated Press version, by Joann Loviglio, begins this way: "In a series of self-portraits he painted to document the progressive ravaging of his brain by Alzheimer's disease, William Utermohlen disappears before our eyes—and his own." The works convey "terror and isolation," "defiance and anger," "shame, confusion and anguish," and "then, in the shadowy final pair of portraits, little more than afterimages of a creative and talented spirit whose identity appears to have vanished." Utermohlen's paintings also appeared in the inaugural issue of the upbeat magazine *Eldr*, which, according to the editorial team, stands for "elder revolution." The cover of this premiere issue, launched in 2007, features a teaser for an article about a 93-year-old sprinter headed to the Senior Olympics and another one for an article on transforming attitudes about aging ("Mad as Hell! Let's Forever Change the Perception of Aging"). The article on Utermohlen is brief and mainly features his remarkable paintings. The caption to one of the paintings, which I prefer to Picasso (and I like Picasso), reads, "The paintings starkly reveal Utermohlen's gradual descent into the ever darkening pit of dementia. At the very least, they are frighteningly poignant. It is almost as if you can see the artist painfully struggling to come out from his foggy reality back into the clarity of his previous self."

Was I looking at the same paintings? I wondered if perhaps Loviglio and the editors at *Eldr* might benefit from lying on a bench in front of Utermohlen's images and looking at them upside down.

15

Duplex Planet

The Art of Conversation

> 🪰 DAVID GREENBERGER: What do you think George Washington's voice
> sounded like?
> FRANK KANSLASKY: Like Jimmy Durante. Who can prove it? Can you
> prove it? No one can. Let it go. Jimmy Durante. Ever hear him
> talk? He didn't sound too bad. You don't want to sound like Tarzan,
> do you?
> DAVID BREWER: It sounded like a dollar bill.
>
> *Duplex Planet*

Some artists take on a single challenge that can shape their entire career. For Rothko, it was color. For Hopper, it was light. David Greenberger has been exploring a single challenge for nearly 30 years—how to portray the individual integrity and humanity of older people he encounters.

Greenberger started his quest in 1979 as an activities director at a nursing home in Boston. He had just received a fine arts degree in painting. On the day he met the residents of Duplex Nursing Home, writes Greenberger, "I abandoned painting. That is to say, I discarded the brushes and canvas, but not the underlying desire to see something in the world around me and then communicate it to others." As an artist, he'd found a new and unexpected medium—the residents of a nursing home. "I wanted others to know these people as I did."

He hasn't given up trying. Greenberger not only has continued to interview older adults but nearly every year he also has produced a unique artifact of those interviews—a graphic novel, a museum exhibit, a periodical, a live performance, a Web site, various musical recordings, documentary films, or radio pieces—that honors the individuality of those who have shared their wisdom with Greenberger. Wisdom isn't a fancy word here. It's not something that separates the "wise man" from the thickheaded masses. To Greenberger, wisdom is simply what comes from knowing a person well enough to recognize his or her unique take on the world. "It comes in the rich language of personal poetics, accidental utterances, and exuberant expressions that are the result of the brain working faster than the mouth."

Greenberger's approach to interviewing is a little unconventional. He devises his questions to disarm his subjects. "What's better, coffee or meat?" Such a question makes you think—about something other than your physical and emotional aches and pains or your fears about aging and dying. Questions like "How close can you get to a penguin?" pull us into the present moment. This isn't oral history. Instead of focusing on who people *were,* Greenberger's questions thrust us into the present and enable us to see who they *are,* and who, if we're lucky enough to survive, we might become. Greenberger plays the jester so that the older men and women he interviews can become ennobled—kings and queens of a world that otherwise largely ignores them.

DAVID GREENBERGER: Who is Frankenstein?

WILLIAM FERGIE FERGUSON: Why he was that theologian, wasn't he? He was supposed to be. Maybe he never appeared as one, but he went and got the name as actually being Frankenstein, but he wasn't. He wasn't nothin', he wasn't of any importance at all, he was just like all of us—a shifter.

FRANCIS MCELROY: He's an outstanding man. I watched him on programs and I think he's an outstanding man and he's liked by several people.

EDGAR MOJOR: He was out of favor, he wasn't a human.

DAVID BREWER: He's a tall bastard.

DAVID GREENBERGER: Can you tell me what a compact disc is?

FRANK KANSLASKY: Who the hell knows! Write this down: Where do you get all these stupid questions? What's a compact disc?! Where do you think we went to school anyway? That's like asking why doesn't snow fall up instead of down. If you look at it long enough it does fall up.

In fact, Greenberger takes a rather sharp turn from oral history. He's interested in fragments rather than whole stories. Fragments of conversations are like intriguing shadow prints of an exchange between people, of a moment shared. "Broken stories and little fragments are a more potent way to get a portrait of the person who is telling it," says Greenberger. "In a complete story, when it is told right, the person telling it almost disappears because the story then takes center stage. A fractured narrative is really about the individual in a more profound way." But those little fragments are what the human brain is conditioned to forget. They are the tidbits the brain bets won't be important in the future and never deeply encodes. After a conversation with a friend, we might associate that moment with a specific piece of information—a restaurant name, for example. Or we might recall a conversation and think, "I really liked that person." But the details of the conversation are gone. Greenberger's obsession is capturing shadow prints of those things we forget about everyday conversations—the ephemeral and sometimes sublime connections between people in the moment.

> DAVID GREENBERGER: Do you have any hobbies?
>
> GERTRUDE CHRISTENSEN: Read, bowl, chase men.
>
> JANE STOCKTON: Coming to dance mostly. And I work crossword puzzles, I'm addicted to that. It keeps your brain more active than most things, even reading. I used to like to read novels, but I've quit that and just read articles now mostly.
>
> FRED SCHAEFER: Usually I don't do very much because I have a problem with my legs, I can't walk. My wife passed away about two years ago and she took my legs with her.
>
> HANNAH LAMONTE: My hobby is breathing right now.

It's easy to misunderstand Greenberger's work. People tend to miss the emphasis on *relationship* when they try to replicate his work. In the wrong hands, it can become a kind of "old people say the darndest things." What is missing in a thin replication of his approach is the time and intensity of relationship building that is the core of his work. What they tend to miss, according to Greenberger is, "how do I really get to know somebody? And how does somebody else really get to know them?" The quirkiness of the questions helped the residents of Duplex Nursing Home (and all the subsequent people Greenberger has talked to) break the traditional rules of decorum. The disarming questions crack open a space in which people can see themselves and each other a little differently. The residents can focus on something outside of themselves and their ailments. "They would wonder, 'Is this guy crazy?' " says Greenberger. And getting them to "wonder[ ] about something outside of themselves felt like one of the few things I could do for them."

Working with people with dementia, Greenberger went even deeper into the moment. William "Fergie" Ferguson, a resident at the Duplex Nursing Home, became his close friend. Greenberger never knew where Fergie was in his mind, and he learned from Fergie that there's no point in correcting seemingly "incorrect" information. Greenberger says, "His belief in it was so complete . . . that it felt like the best way to continue spending time with him in those moments was to ask him about this thing that I knew never happened." It wasn't about the data. It was about the time they spent together. So maybe Fergie never hung out with Eisenhower. But the way he talked very much reflected who he was—he had been an insurance salesman who talked to people for a living.

Be where they are. Nothing quite demonstrates the wisdom of that deceptively simple phrase than a story Greenberger told me about a man he met in a nursing home in Portland, Oregon. He'd been hired to do a project with a variety of people who lived in independent living centers and visited meal sites and day centers. At one facility, staff members were eager for Greenberger to meet a man who loved to talk. He'd had a serious brain injury of some kind, a tumor perhaps, and the shape of his skull was changed. He was in a wheelchair. He stayed active, said Greenberger, "by going up and down the hallway, pulling himself ahead with one leg, his one working leg." He was happy to talk to Greenberger and would humor him by answering any questions he had about anything. "And then," says Greenberger, "we would get to the end of the hallway and he would turn around and he would have to meet me all over again. He had no idea who I was." So they developed a rhythm together. "It wasn't my rhythm, but it was the rhythm I had to do if I wanted to be with him. Walking up and down the hall, I say hello again, and we start over."

Greenberger acknowledges that his hallway rhythm might be harder for the man's friends and family, who would find it difficult to shed the image of who he *was* to fully embrace who he *is*. But Greenberger knew no background. "I think that is one of the things that would benefit people—to meet people as they are."

Do people get that from his work? "When somebody gets it, they really get it," says Greenberger. But sometimes they don't. And that, Greenberger thinks, reflects a lot about their attitudes about aging and dying. "When they say it's depressing, what they are really saying is 'I don't want to know about declining—don't show me this.'"

The early years of Duplex Planet (1979–90) were focused on periodicals, little booklets with photos, artwork, and bits of dialogues and monologues of the older people Greenberger interviewed. But in addition to being a visual artist, Greenberger is also a musician and performer. In the early 1990s, he began to perform selected fragments that he'd collected—sometimes in a lecture format, sometimes collaborating with other artists to set them to music. In 1995, he created a spoken word performance called *1001 Real Apes* with the Boston-based Birdsongs of the Mesozoic, which they recorded on CD some 10 years later. By 2007, Greenberger had made more than a dozen CDs from the project, including several featuring songs that he produced based on the lyrics of Duplex resident Ernest Noyes Brookings and that were played by an eclectic array of bands from across the United States.

In 2006, Greenberger interviewed older residents of East Los Angeles and worked with musicians from the band Los Lobos to envelop the interviews in music. But in general, he prefers reading the words of the people he meets in his own distinct voice. "As soon as some people hear an old person's voice they think, 'it's an old documentary thing, I've heard that before, I'm bored.'" He makes a sharp turn to avoid such easy dismissal. His radio pieces aren't "a souvenir of these people's lives." Instead, by putting them into someone else's voice, he hopes people will glean a common experience of aging.

Something has happened in the years that Greenberger has been practicing the art of conversation. In the beginning, he was a quirky, art-world phenomenon. When I first read the *Duplex Planet* book in 1994, I laughed until I cried. Weak with laughter and weeping, I kept turning the pages. When I had time to reflect, I worried about what had struck me as so funny. Was I laughing *at?* Or *with?* When I reread the book and newsletters now, a laugh still bursts out unexpectedly. But I don't worry anymore whether Greenberger facilitated years of laughter at the expense of the people he interviews. That jolt of laughter comes from a deep appreciation for the wit and emotions he ignites. The longevity of the project has given it gravitas. Greenberger's periodicals, books, CDs, radio spots, and art exhibits have become playful, earnest, and lasting tributes to their sources.

Thirty years is a long time to do a project. Now in his 50s, Greenberger definitely sees things in a different way. "It seems like yesterday that my daughter was in kindergarten and now she's in college, and when I telescope this ahead, I'm going to be dead." He doesn't say this with fear, but like he's facing a mystery. When his daughter came home from college for a visit with a friend, he thought, "Wow—I realized she is meeting the people she is going to know after I'm dead. I picture this really clearly—her calling up a friend and saying 'My Dad died.'" He

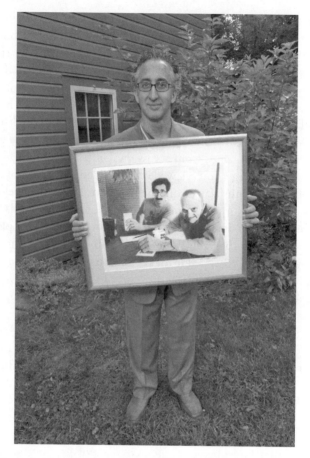

David Greenberger with a younger self and Ernest Noyes Brookings.
Photo by Joe Putrock.

was comforted by the thought in a way. She was out meeting the people who would support her after he was gone. And they were good people.

Greenberger's work has enjoyed some mainstream recognition. *Rolling Stone* did an article on him; he recently appeared on the show *Life Part 2*; and the book jacket of *Duplex Planet: Everybody's Asking Who I Was* features blurbs from magicians Penn & Teller, director Jonathan Demme, and musician Lou Reed, who calls the book "One of life's little wonders." As the *New York Times* said of the book, "The tales of the Duplex . . . are modern-day versions of Chaucer's reports from the road to Canterbury; they resonate with a wry humor and startling insight."

But I think we still have a ways to go before Greenberger's lesson is fully absorbed by the general public. Be where they are. Concentrate on the sublime and ephemeral moments of a conversation. And let the brain go faster than the mouth. Perhaps these should be written into a handbook distributed far and wide: "The Art of Conversation." We at the Center on Age and Community are making an effort to capture and disseminate the essence of Greenberger's approach by documenting the arc of his career on film. We expect the film to be completed in spring 2009.

DAVID GREENBERGER: Where do manners come from?

FERGIE: Comes from your inner soul. I don't mean your ass, your inner soul, s-o-u-l.

FERGIE: What are those, all-wool socks?

DAVID GREENBERGER: No, acrylic.

FERGIE: He was a good boy, acrylic, too bad he died.

FERGIE: Where do you come from, Connecticut?

DAVID GREENBERGER: Erie, Pennsylvania.

FERGIE: Oh, that's the wet part of Pennsylvania.

DAVID GREENBERGER: Have you ever been there?

FERGIE: I've been to Erie, but not when it's wet.

DAVID GREENBERGER: Are there enough legal holidays? If not, what's missing?

VILJO LEHTO: My birthday should be a legal holiday—why not? I'm a human, ain't I?

DAVID GREENBERGER: What's the easiest job in the world?

ERNEST MARTIN: Beg pardon?

DAVID GREENBERGER: What's the easiest job in the world?

ERNEST MARTIN: The easiest?

DAVID GREENBERGER: Job.

ERNEST MARTIN: Job?

DAVID GREENBERGER: Yeah, in the world.

ERNEST MARTIN: Bein' a politician I think.

DAVID GREENBERGER: What's the easiest job in the world?

THEODORE BARRIEN: That's a tough one, I don't know. I can tell you the hardest job, bein' good all the time! (*chuckles*)

16

The Photography of Wing Young Huie

🐦 Other than my children, nobody comes to visit us. Nobody. Not a friend that we knew all those years in line dancing, bowling, families that we vacationed with. All those people are gone.

Gil

A Vietnamese Elvis impersonator. A "redneck" Chinese restaurant owner near the Okefenokee swamp. Two Latina school girls giggling on an unmade bed under the watchful eyes of fuzzy stuffed animals nailed to the wall above them. The luminous face of Shalemar Flying Horse, a young woman bundled in a blue-black parka on a gray Minneapolis winter day, dwarfed by a circle of tall boys in blue-black parkas who surround her.

These are the photographs by Wing Young Huie. Trained as a print journalist, Huie taught himself photography. About 15 years ago, he set down his notepad and started following people around with cameras exclusively. A second-generation Chinese American from Duluth, Minnesota, Huie is drawn to photographing people and places that don't fit into the apple pie image of the United States of America. Huie wandered around Frogtown, one of the oldest neighborhoods in St. Paul and home to the largest Hmong community in Minnesota, for several years. He exhibited his work in a vacant lot in Frogtown on makeshift gallery walls covered in plastic sheeting to protect them from the weather.

Huie eventually expanded beyond Frogtown to photograph multiple neighborhoods that border Lake Street—a major artery through which courses the lifeblood of some of the most diverse neighborhoods of the Twin Cities. Huie photographed for 4 years; the result was a stunning six-mile long exhibit of 675 photographs that appeared in store windows, bus stops, and the sides of buildings. Huie negotiated with 150 businesses to show the work, which ranged from 8 by 12 inches to 8 by 12 feet. In 2001, Huie and his wife, Tara, embarked on a road trip across the United States to explore the country through the eyes of Asian Americans. *Nine Months in America: An Ethnocentric Tour* was commissioned by the Minnesota Museum of American Art in St. Paul, and the show, featuring 105 photographs as well as video, premiered there in April 2004.

Then in 2006, Huie was awarded the first residency in applied arts from the University of Wisconsin–Milwaukee's Center on Age and Community. For 3 months, an artist interested in exploring the topic of aging and dementia could do just that. It was a rare opportunity for an artist to think deeply and to experiment to find out what works—and, of course, what doesn't work. In his first month in Milwaukee, Huie experienced a steep learning curve. Assisted living. Long-term care. Adult day care. HUD housing. Skilled nursing. Family care. Alzheimer's Association. Title 19. He worried a bit about how he could show the depth of the everyday experience of living with dementia. "And then I realized, why should this be any different? I backed off the word 'dementia.' I was thinking of these people as being *different*. Since I haven't spent that much time in senior communities, walking in seemed strange. But it doesn't take long before you get used to it, and you start to see individuals better, and personalities. In the end, the process was similar to my other projects."

Over the 3 months of his residency, he photographed and interviewed five constellations of people across a wide spectrum of symptoms, stages, and backgrounds. These are their stories, in words and images.

Minnie and Granddaughter Nina

Huie explained why he had wanted to photograph Minnie:

> I'm just drawn to certain people when I walk into a room as a photographer, and I don't really know what that is. With Minnie, who wouldn't want to photograph her? She was apart from the group. She has such an engaging smile. When she's not smiling, she seems to be in her own world. There was something about that that really intrigued me. The way her hair was braided, it was so thoughtful. I photographed her in her church. She's wearing a white coat with her white hair and white shoes, and she's holding a white Bible. I took a close-up of the white Bible with her red fingernails.

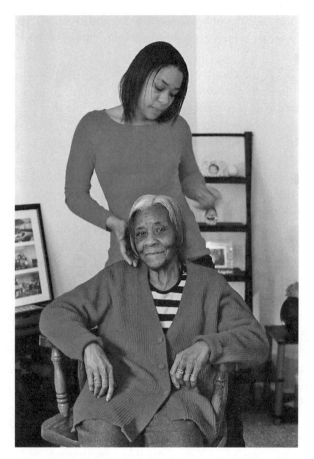

Minnie and Nina, 2007. Photo by Wing Young Huie.

Nina offers family background:

> I'm 25 and my grandmother lives with me. Her ID says she was born in '22, but she likes to say she's sixteen. . . .
>
> She is very healthy. Her memory is OK, but she remembers only the good things. You know, when you have terrible things happen in your life you just block it out. They say twice a child, you know. How you come in this world is how you go out of this world.
>
> I think it's unusual that someone young like me is taking care of an elderly person. It's a huge responsibility. When she goes to sleep every night she sees me. When she wakes up she sees me. Every day. Nobody wanted

to step up and do it. I'm not getting paid or whatever. I just do what I love. It can be very frustrating, but I'm fine with it. I don't know. You just got to follow your heart.

Huie recorded the following conversation among Nina, her grand-mother, and him:

NINA: The South was really racist, with white people saying "nigger." How did that make you feel as a person?

MINNIE: Back in those days they did call you "nigger." When I heard that word I paid them no attention.

NINA: I think that's good. Because I talk to a lot of elderly people and usually that is a big issue with them. They went through a lot, with white people just degrading them.

MINNIE: A lot of people still do that.

. . .

NINA: Does it bother you that you don't remember everything?

MINNIE: No, because you can't remember everything. I don't remember nothing bad.

HUIE: Why do you think that is?

MINNIE: Because they love you more when you're kind and loving.

Gil and Vic

Huie is accustomed to telling stories of migration, capturing the jour-ney of how people get to where they are. He was fascinated with Vic and Gil, who grew up a block away from each other on Milwaukee's South Side and live there still. In many ways they've stayed still while their deep circle of friends have migrated away from them. Gil invited Huie into his home to photograph him and his wife. As he crossed the thresh-old, Gil told him that he was the first to do so in many, many months. Huie asked Gil how they first met:

Three of us had just come home from the war in 1946 and we decided to go the Dreamland Ballroom in the far north side of Milwaukee. This pretty little blonde-haired gal came dancing by. She was standing with a group of 10, 12 girls from the factory where she worked, shooting the breeze. You talk about love at first sight. It was a feeling I can't even express. It was over-whelming. Don't ask me, I have no idea how I had the guts to go and ask her for a dance.

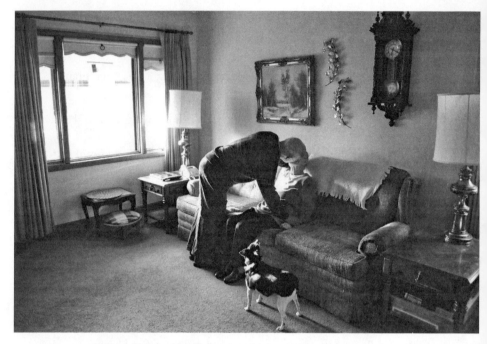

Vic and Gil, 2007. Photo by Wing Young Huie.

Later, in the lounge we both had a Coca-Cola and I got a nickel back in change. I kept that nickel, and later she put it on a chain. We found out we were both Polish Catholics and lived on the South Side within walking distance. That night I gave her a quick kiss, just a little peck on the cheek, and all the home way it bothered me. I was too bold. I should have been more of a gentleman.

. . .

On Saturday nights we watch Lawrence Welk. If one of our favorite songs comes on we'll dance, cheek to cheek. She can still do the polka.

I hope that more couples could experience the kind of marriage Vic and I have had. We raised three wonderful children. We belonged to a couples bowling league, did country line dancing in three different places every week. One day when we were dancing, I noticed that people who were good dancers would slowly move away and avoid her. Then the manager at the bowling alley told me, "I don't know if you're aware but some of the people on the teams are not pleased with the way Vic is bowling." For a bowling team, your average is important for winning first place and all that stuff.

So I gave up the bowling and dancing. Slowly all these things ended. Friends weren't coming to the house anymore. Other than my children, nobody comes to visit us. Nobody. Not a friend that we knew all those years in line dancing, bowling, families that we vacationed with. All those people are gone.

Why? I guess that's normal with most people who end up in wheelchairs or oxygen tanks. Their friends slowly feel that it's either holding them back or it hurts them to see them disabled or they're embarrassed. It really hurts. I lie in bed and think about it.

Alfred Yao and Huifen Lin

Huie notes that "Judy Chin is the daughter of Alfred Yao and Huifen Lin, who has Alzheimer's. Alfred and Huifen moved in with Judy and her husband after she was diagnosed. Judy did most of the talking. Alfred speaks English but it's sometimes hard to understand."

My dad is originally from China and then went to Taiwan in 1949 and then immigrated to the United States. He was in the Chinese air force in the Second War, against the Japanese who attacked China.

My mom, before she got Alzheimer's disease, was very sharp. She never used the telephone address book. She could remember everything in her head. My dad really wanted to take her to see the world, but then she became sick. My dad tried all the ways, the American way, Chinese herbal medicines, just trying to help her. Maybe there will be a special cure, some magic, something will happen.

It was difficult for him to accept that my mom will not get better. For the 57 years they have been together he has always been devoted to her. They used to listen to Chinese opera and dance together. My dad taught himself to play the erhu, a two-stringed Chinese instrument. He will play love songs on the erhu every day to comfort her and bring back some of the special moments they had before.

There's a Chinese saying that when the parents have been sick for a long time you won't have good children anymore. Before, I would feel guilty about going places, but now I feel that I can only do my best and that I have to live my own life. My dad understands that we will always be here to help.

. . .

My dad is old country way. We will try to keep our mom as long as possible. But we're concerned that dad takes care of himself because he spends all his time taking care of mom. I think our cultural obligation is changing.

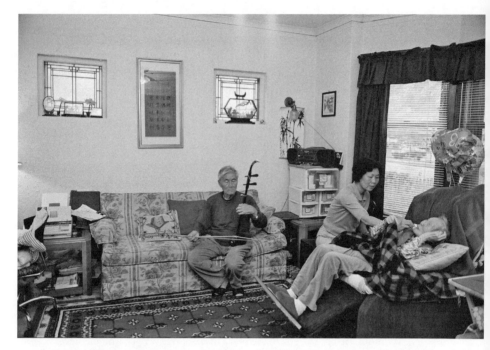

Alfred Yao and Huifen Lin and Judy Chin, 2007. Photo by Wing Young Huie.

Even in Taiwan people are moving away from home to a different city and have their own lives and cannot take care of their parents. So they hire out workers from other countries like Vietnam or the Philippines to come in to help out. The children will chip in money to hire them.

Alfred had this to say:

I never feel angry. When I feel sad, I play music, and then I'm happy.

Everybody is going to be old. It's the nature of things. I never worry about it. If you don't think about it, you'll always feel young. I always think positive thoughts.

Lucia and Her Daughter Juana

Huie interviewed Juana and her mother, Lucia.

My mom is almost 90 years old. We have a big family. She has 11 children and 48 grandchildren. She's a happy old lady. She likes to sing [and] play the guitar. She goes to church every Sunday. She likes to sew her own dolls.

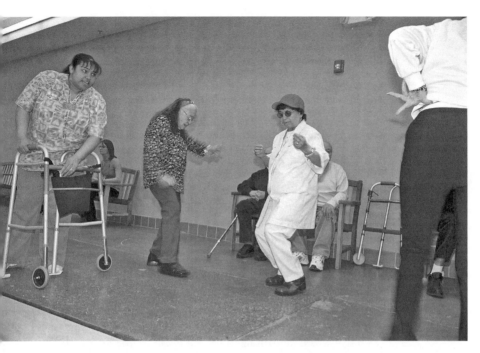

Lucia and her daughter Juanita dance together at the United Community
Center in Milwaukee. Photo by Wing Young Huie.

She likes to talk too much (*laughs*). She likes to tell old stories from the
past growing up in Puerto Rico. She was 48 when she had me. She had long
white hair and was old, so I thought she was my grandmother. I didn't realize she was my mother until first grade.

Her mom first put her in school when she was 10. A lot of people did
that. They put her in first grade, with all the little kids. Because she was so
much bigger than the other kids they called her names. Nobody wanted to
play with her. They said that she had lice. So she rolled up a rug and hit
them. She fought back all the time. So finally her mother took her out of
school. So she never finished first grade.

She says that she wishes that she had stayed in school and maybe
gone to college. She doesn't know numbers. She can only count to 10.
She can't read music but she taught herself to play guitar. She plays all
the time. I can hear her through the floor playing and singing in her bed-
room. She says that her age is not too heavy for her. She means it doesn't
bother her.

Florence and Ronny

Florence recounts Ronny's life:

> Ronny is 62 years old, born in Norwood, Massachusetts. We learned when he was 6 years old that he had Down's syndrome. There was no education . . . in the public schools in Massachusetts at that time if you were retarded. So the Sisters of St. Francis in Wisconsin offered [to] our archbishop to open up a school in Massachusetts for the retarded. We entered Ronny there when he was 6 years old. He was there for 10 years, living with the nuns. They said he was an A student. He learned to read well and read the newspaper all his life until this dementia happened.
>
> My husband was in charge of a 90-acre farm hospital school in Canton, Massachusetts. He hired Ronny, and he was a good employee for 34 years working with the grounds crew. To this day all the fellows think the world of him. He was voted employee of the year 3 years before he retired in 2000. That was from a staff of over 300 teachers, doctors, and nurses and so forth. He made us very proud.
>
> He was doing fine until last winter around Christmastime when he began to forget where some things were and began to lose his way. It became hard for me to take care of him. It changed his personality. I never heard him swear. Now he curses and wants to hit the nurse. He was the nicest fellow. He liked to talk about sports. He won't even watch television. Every week we would watch the Patriots, Red Sox, Bruins, and Celtics on Direct TV. Now he'll pull out the wires. He doesn't seem like he wants to live. Ronnie is 62, so this must be the way the Lord wants to take him. I wish he would take him and not make him suffer.
>
> He's now at the Lutheran Home. I lived with him all my life. It's like giving up your best friend. I couldn't live with him because you ache and you cry. You feel stress all the time. He wouldn't take his pills. He wouldn't eat or drink. His mind that was Ronnie Dodge is gone. It's a different mind that is in him now.

Huie took nearly 3,000 photographs during his 3-month residency in Milwaukee. He made double prints of every photograph he took and gave one to the people he photographed. He also gave his subjects a chance to shoot back. Part of Huie's original concept for the residency was to explore turning over the tools of the trade to the people he was photographing. In some of the more intimate settings, when Huie was shooting one on one with couples in their homes, asking them to pho-

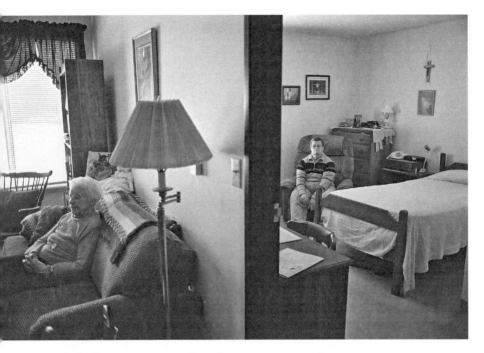

Florence and Ronny, 2007. Photo by Wing Young Huie.

tograph their own lives felt too intrusive and demanding. Huie chose instead to give cameras to two of the adult day programs through which
he had met Lucia and Minnie, the United Community Center (UCC)
and the Good Shepherd House.

Huie didn't want to impose any rules on the photographers. He selected simple, film-based (not digital) point-and-shoot cameras and gave
them to the staff of the day centers to distribute to their participants.
Staff members simply asked participants if they wanted to try it. If someone said yes, he or she got a camera. At UCC, day-care manager Nelva
Olin took participants on a tour through the building. They clicked
everything; each other, the staff, the building itself. For some, holding a
camera was a completely new experience. "It makes me feel rich!" said
one woman, who had never used a camera before. At Good Shepherd
House, day-care coordinator Marcia Hochstetter said she was surprised by
who picked up the camera. "Jim took pictures almost all day," said
Hochstetter, "and he usually sleeps most of the time he's here." Inspired
by the response to the exercise, Huie aims to try it again on a larger scale,

to study how and why it works, and to share the results in a training manual.

Huie hopes to exhibit the work as part of a show that would tour museums. But he's not done photographing yet. "I think I just scratched the surface. I'd like to get a more national perspective. I'd also like to photograph in my hometown," he said. "I think because I'm 52, issues of aging seem more real to me now."

Autobiographies by People with Dementia

> ✦ And identity is funny being yourself is funny as you are never your-
> self to yourself except as you remember yourself and then of course
> you do not believe yourself. That is really the trouble with an auto-
> biography you do not of course you do not really believe yourself
> why should you, you know so well so very well that it is not yourself,
> it could not be yourself because you cannot remember right and if
> you do not remember right it does not sound right and of course it
> does not sound right because it is not right. You are of course never
> yourself.
>
> Gertrude Stein

Identity is a rich blend of individual personality and the people, places, and things you encounter, who and which in turn shape you. Writing, whether fiction or curly-lettered journal entries, gives you a chance to stop the spinning for a few minutes, to take control and pin down who you think you are by leaving an artifact. Unless you are Gertrude Stein, who prefers to keep spinning. Writing maps our journey of becoming. As Stein suggests, we never actually arrive. We never *are* ourselves. We are always becoming ourselves—even in the depths of dementia.

Writing is a powerful tool for people with dementia and for the spouse, children, and friends who are partnered with them in their care. It enables people with dementia to order their thoughts and share them without the usual markings of the disease. "You won't see a picture of me in this book putting my shirt on inside out," writes Richard Taylor in his book *Alzheimer's from the Inside Out.* "It happens many times a week. You won't hear me fishing for a word, because I have time to pause when writing. You won't see me wandering around, not knowing or car-ing where I am. I look and sound 'normal.'" Writing can act as a mask that lets people with dementia elude stigma. In the chat rooms of the

Dementia Advocacy and Support Network International (DASNI), it can be hard to tell who has dementia and who doesn't. Through writing, people with dementia have the choice to reveal their illness rather than have their illness reveal them.

For friends and family of people with dementia, writing provides a way to channel stressful emotions. Writing also gives them a way to piece together what they see as falling apart—the history and personality of a loved one with dementia. There are many, many published stories of this kind. Most commonly, these stories give some structure to the fear and powerlessness caregivers feel. Sue Miller writes: "Along the way, while I was working on what I hoped would be my useful memoir—reconstructing my father again for myself, imagining him whole, putting together the pieces that slowly disintegrated and broke off—I found there were still things I could learn from him, still things he could teach me, things that helped bring him home in my own memory from the faraway land of his disease."

Biography and memoirs are, of course, primarily about the subject or writer and his or her experience. John Bayley's *Elegy for Iris,* for example, is primarily about John Bayley's efforts to understand his relationship to one of the great writers and thinkers of our time as she experienced Alzheimer's disease.

Autobiographies by people with dementia open a whole other window into the experience of the disease—the struggle to tell and track over time one's story in the first person. The number of "memoirs" by people with dementia is growing. Robert Davis's *My Journey into Alzheimer's Disease* (1989) and Diana Friel McGowin's *Living in the Labyrinth* (1993) were written when advocacy was done almost exclusively by caregivers and researchers and when the Alzheimer's Association was still solidifying its national network and working hard to raise awareness and provide support services. Davis, a minister, relates his spiritual struggles with Alzheimer's. McGowin's story, told in a generous and quirky voice, is one of overcoming enormous self-doubt to find the strength to tell family and friends of her disease.

After forerunners Davis and McGowin came a second round of autobiographies, including Cary Henderson's *Partial View* (1998), Larry Rose's *Show Me the Way to Go Home* (1995), Christine Bryden's *Who Will I Be When I Die?* (1998), and Thomas DeBaggio's *Losing My Mind* (2002). These books emerged when the Alzheimer's Association had transformed from a group of passionate volunteers into a professional organization.

Services, like 24-hour call lines, support groups, and SAFE Return, were solidified. The first medications (cholinesterase inhibitors) were becoming available. There was hope in both care and treatment. This group of authors with dementia achieved the field's version of "rock star" status. Bryden's book developed an international following; she went on to publish a second book (*Dancing with Dementia* [2005]) and to become the subject of a documentary film. DeBaggio appeared on *Oprah* and on multiple episodes of NPR's *All Things Considered.* A documentary film crew followed DeBaggio for a bit as well, but, as he told me in an interview, they seemed disappointed when he didn't die within the arc of their storyline, and they dropped the project. Like Bryden, DeBaggio wrote a second book, *When It Gets Dark: An Enlightened Reflection on a Life with Alzheimer's* (2003), and a third that went unpublished. This was a new era. Clearly, there was a growing interest in hearing the voices of people with dementia.

I had mixed feelings about this phase of the "dementia autobiography" movement. Advancements in scanning technology were making it easier for doctors to diagnose dementia, particularly Alzheimer's disease, earlier and earlier. People could get an answer to the question that haunted them: "Is this forgetfulness normal? Or is it . . . ?" In every case, these authors had early diagnosis and early onset—all were under 65 when they were diagnosed. Early onset represents a thin sliver of the Alzheimer's experience, well under 10 percent of all cases. With the new diagnostic category of "mild cognitive impairment," some people will receive a diagnosis that might never "translate" into Alzheimer's. The story of Alzheimer's that came out of the second wave of autobiographies by authors with early onset was of a person deeply engaged in family (sometimes with children still at home), work, and community. Disability and death at their age are still relatively rare, and one of the core themes in the books is the sudden awareness of mortality. DeBaggio's *Losing My Mind,* in particular, seems weighted more toward the shock of his mortality at what he sees as the height of his career than a description of the actual symptoms of his condition.

On the other hand, the Alzheimer's disease movement needed a jolt. At the turn of the twenty-first century, it was still "speaking for" people with Alzheimer's. The board of the Alzheimer's Association wouldn't have a person with dementia sitting on it until 2008. As of this writing, the organization has put together task forces and holds town hall meetings with people in the early stages to help guide them in providing services to meet the unique needs of this group. These autobiographies were also powerful because dementia was, and still is, too often written off as something that just happens when you get old (and, the logic goes, when you will be dying soon anyway), which makes it hard to mobilize policy changes for support of people living with the condition.

I was also a little leery of the dementia autobiographies because of the form they took. These texts seemed uniquely positioned to challenge America's obsession with the independent, rugged individual. The authors were in a position to imagine and depict an interdependent self in complex ways. But, instead, they were all pretty standard "I" stories. "I" was this person. I got diagnosed. I now struggle with these symptoms. Here is how I hope to live out my days. The authors usually hid the acknowledgment of the help they received from editors and cowriters in the preface, footnotes, or epilogue. They wrote to repair their "I." And I can't blame them. The "relational self" doesn't receive much credit in our culture. American culture has a hard time understanding collaboration. Part of the reason is legal. Who gets copyright credit for a collaboratively written piece? Part of the reason is our strong focus on the individual. We think that this must be some *one's* story. Americans tend to think that people are either independent or dependent—we can't possibly be in between. We like black or white. We don't do well with gray.

One of the latest entries into the field of Alzheimer's rendered in the first person is Richard Taylor's *Alzheimer's from the Inside Out* (2006). I heard Richard speak in Atlanta at the Dementia Care Conference in September 2006. I'd been receiving e-mails from him for some time. These e-mails, which went out to a long list of people, were impressively pestilent. This man was angry and frustrated, with doctors, with well-meaning friends and acquaintances, with the disease, with the organizations that were designed to "help" him, with the culture in which he was experiencing this disease. His signature lines at the bottom of the e-mails dared people who shared his feelings to act:

Stand up! Speak Up! Do not become a victim
    of your own silence.
Speak for yourself and those who will follow. Ask Carers and Friends to do
    the same.
Today will never be here again. Time is of the Essence!! Use it wisely!!!
Tell as many people as possible your
perceptions of your interactions with

professionals, with carers, with friends, with
strangers, with your government.
They won't change unless they know, and
they can't know unless and until you
SPEAK UP!
Seek to create a Palpable Sense of Change
and of Urgency!
Join a Crusade, Now!
Be a Crusader, Now!
Lead a Crusade, Now!
"Aim above morality.
Be not simply good,
Be good for something."

Henry David Thoreau

As a retired professor of psychology diagnosed with "probable" Alzheimer's, he was uniquely qualified to rage against the machine. I had seen other conferences that sought out the opinions of people with dementia, and it always seemed a bit like a polite sideshow. The audience would listen attentively, encourage the speakers, wait for wisdom, and hope it would all go smoothly. But did people with dementia really have insights to give? Were the members of the audience really engaging with them as experts? Or listening politely until a time when they could wrestle with the tough questions of the field? I was eager to hear Richard because I thought he might break through this veil of politeness. And that he did.

When you mention Richard's name now, eyebrows go up. It's as if he has spilled his emotions and made a mess of the Alzheimer's scene. He writes angry e-mails to the CEO of the Alzheimer's Association, daring him to fund psychosocial research. Richard has forgotten—or perhaps ignores—the rules of decorum. He is not a victim holding on to hope for a cure. He is an activist. He is an activist with "probable" Alzheimer's.

Compared to his e-mails though, Richard's book is rather tame. Perhaps the book contains his emotions in a format in which social rules are understood and followed. The collection of short essays are simultaneously insightful, sardonic, and warmly funny. They capture and cut through the broken systems of diagnosis and care for people with dementia with precision and wit. They look deep into the dynamics of doctors, families, and friendships and offer earnest suggestions for changing the attitudes and behaviors of all parties—himself included.

Like the narrators of all other first-person stories of dementia, Taylor explains that writing helps him not only to understand himself, but to *have* a self. "Writing has become a confirmation to me, of me, and by me. Some people believe 'they think therefore they are.' I write, therefore I am." While Taylor shares this mission with all other Alzheimer's autobiographers, his writing steps in a new direction. He dares to question whether the emperor is clothed, to question the labeling and diagnostic guidelines for a disease that is confirmable only by autopsy. "The more I read about scientific breakthroughs in the basic research on Alzheimer's disease, the more I'm convinced that lacking a complete, well-documented, and universally accepted map of the mind and how a healthy mind works ensures we cannot yet identify the root cause of the disease of dementia. If we don't know how something works, how can we fix it? How will we know it is fixed?" A page later, he writes: "From my perspective as a person living with the diagnosis, there is far too much emphasis on the label, the name, and the symptoms generally associated with the disease and too little emphasis on the individuals who actually have the disease."

Taylor's doppelgänger from the medical perspective is Peter Whitehouse, whose *The Myth of Alzheimer's* also questions the labeling of Alzheimer's as a single, specific disease. Whitehouse writes: "Alzheimer's is a hundred-year old myth that is over the hill. The entire scientific, technological, and political framework for aging needs to be reassessed to better serve patients and families in order to help people maximize their quality of life as they move along the path of cognitive aging."

Taylor offers us perceptive suggestions to accomplish just that. He points to several aspects of the disease experience that need more research, including fear: "I believe our fears, and specifically my fears—fear of losing control, fear of what will happen tomorrow, fear of who I will become, fear of the unknown, and the list goes on—are as much or more of a problem for me in my day-to-day living than is the disease itself." Later he addresses fear again: "Specifically for me, someone with Alzheimer's disease, fear is the 3,000-pound elephant tromping around in my mind. If I ignore it and pretend it isn't there, I do so at my own risk. I have never learned how to train this elephant. Now that it has suddenly grown 1,000-fold, I fear it is out of control and frankly beyond control!"

Taylor's book provides many insights into the experience of dementia, but perhaps the most courageous and insightful thing that Taylor does in his book is reject the black and white view of aging and dementia. Half full or half empty? Taylor throws out the glass. "Finally, after 62 years of living, I am beginning to see the gray in life's experience as the heart of the experience." He continues: "I am an extension of my family, and they are an extension of me. Forget this half-full / half-empty stuff—it is as useful as asking me if I am a Pentium 3 or a Pentium 4."

Taylor revisits the appeal of "gray" thinking later in the book when he wrestles with being perceived as an object rather than a subject, an "it" rather than a "thou." "So how do you relate to a Thou who does not act or think like Thou?" he asks. "I don't have a solution. I don't want it to happen to me. Just on my own, I don't know how to avoid it. I do know that I continue to need to be recognized as a Thou, to have my personhood recognized. Please understand, I am still here."

The hardest thing about dementia for families is undoubtedly coming to some terms with the changes in their loved one and at the same time the constancy—the presence that is still there. Half full or half empty? Independent or dependent? Where do I end and the perceptions of me begin? How can we pin down the "push me-pull me" of the self? Is it possible in a country that so clearly comes down on the side of the individual able to slip on those boots and pull himself or herself up by their straps? Taylor shakes his fists at the very notion that the distinction matters: "I am no longer who I formerly was. I am no longer like everyone, but there is still a good deal of me left. Am I half empty or half full? What difference does it make in terms of being a full and equal member of the family? It's tough for everyone! My heart aches and I want to shout: 'I'm a different Thou, not a quarter It and three quarters Thou.'"

Richard Taylor is the first in a new wave of activists with dementia. Technology, research incentives, and public education are enabling doctors to diagnose Alzheimer's and other dementias earlier and earlier. As more and more people receive these early diagnoses, we will no doubt witness the creation of an army of advocates who will fight for the rights of people with cognitive disability, however they might be officially diagnosed (or not diagnosed). The traditional, published autobiography is just one tool that this new generation of advocates has at their disposal. There are a growing number of organizations (and Web sites) run *by* people with dementia *for* people with dementia. Thus far, these groups have primarily focused on giving the newly diagnosed safe harbor. People with symptoms give advice to each other over the Internet or at conferences and workshops. Those without symptoms are invited to join the discussion to learn about the experience from those living it. In November 2007, the Alzheimer's Association launched a Web site *for* people in early stages, and DASNI has started to envision advocacy on a larger scale, hoping to push politicians to declare dementia a global health concern. Alzheimer's Spoken Here (www.ash.org), which features a blog for people with dementia, is moving toward practical issues; working, for example, with design students at Columbia College in Chicago to design a more accessible computer keyboard.

The authors of the early narratives of dementia have a common purpose. In their own way, each explains what drove them to write. "Perhaps understanding the 'blackness' and 'lost' feelings," writes Robert Davis in 1989, "will help families to be more understanding of the unreasonable actions they must deal with." Diana McGowin defines herself almost purely in terms of her usefulness to society and has a heightened awareness of her loss of social value when she must stop working—so much so that she replaces her paid work with writing the memoir in hopes that it will be of use to others going through the disease. Like McGowin and Davis, Cary Henderson sees writing as a way he can help other people, a way he can make some sense out of what seems a senseless disease. "I'm taking it as one of my duties," he writes, "to sort of get people with Alzheimer's knowledgeable about what they can expect and what they can do, and of course, what they can't do." All three writers crave being of use. They write through their disease, sharing their thoughts and feelings as a way to help others on the same journey.

The new generation of dementia activists builds on the foundation laid by Davis, McGowin, Henderson, and others. While the earlier narratives looked inward, the more recent writings, including blog entries and Taylor's missives, turn outward. Stepping into the path forged by the disability rights movement(s), these writers look to make the world a more hospitable place for people with dementia. Mary Ann Becklenberg is such a person. I met Mary Ann, who has early onset and is in the early stages of dementia, at the Dementia Care Conference in 2007, when we spoke on a panel together. She talked passionately about her experiences, particularly about her fears of being found out—of slipping up in conversations and hiding her misunderstandings and confusion under her smooth social graces. Then, all of a sudden, she paused: "I'm going to say something new here that I haven't thought of before. I think maybe I'm going to try not to think of myself as the center of the universe all the time. I don't think people really care if I say the wrong thing. Think of what I can do if I don't worry about that all the time!"

The bravery of Taylor's book, and of Mary Ann's sudden realization, is to be found in the insistence on looking outward—toward fixing the culture that surrounds and shapes the dementia experience, a culture on which these activists' actions can have tremendous impact. Their words and their actions tell us indisputably: they are and always will be *more* than their dementia.

> Some days, I'm not easy to talk to. Most days, I'm not easy to listen to. I have an ability to say in a thousand words what many other people could say in 10 words. That isn't to say I'm not funny, clever, interesting, and worth listening to. It's just a fact that, even on good days, I talk too much.
>
> . . .
>
> Daily, I say to myself, "What's the big deal? So what if you are losing some of your independence and are swallowing more dependence? You thought you were going to be the first human being not to grow old?"
>
> . . .
>
> Thank heavens for Dr. Alzheimer. He was the first to begin to understand me, or at least to understand me when I was dead. Now I am working on the alive part of the understanding me in a joint venture with my caregivers.

Conclusion

How and Why to Move through
Our Fears about Dementia

People fear the lack of control that dementia entails. But taking control of attitudes and care systems *now* can help us shape the experience of dementia for those now and in the future. What specifically do we need to remember and do to improve the cultural experience of living with memory loss? Scientists should certainly keep working on prevention. But here is a synopsis of the kind of culture work we—all of us, people with dementia, their families, their friends, their professional care partners, even those without direct relationship to someone with dementia—can do *right now* to create better lives for people with dementia.

1. Insist on Complex Stories of Dementia

We need to tell and ought to expect to hear more complicated stories of memory loss than we are commonly fed in mainstream media. Stories of loss and emotional pain are part of the dementia experience. Those going through the experience of dementia need to tell these stories to share their pain with their families and friends. But the experience of dementia is more than the stories of loss and pain—it is bigger than a tightly told tragedy can capture. Dementia as an individual and societal tragedy is a tempting story to tell. It is big and scary and can motivate people to call and urge their senators to support more funding for research. Tragic stories can motivate people to call the Alzheimer's Association and donate money for support services. Money for scientific research and money for care are both good things. Some of the researchers I interviewed for this book were adamant in their belief that raising public awareness of Alzheimer's disease is more important than the tone of that message. But there are real costs to the tragedies crowding out more balanced stories. High-pitched tragic stories that scare us by depicting Alzheimer's and other dementias as an existential horror, as devoid of any meaning or purpose, can paralyze us. People panic over normal, age-related memory loss. Care partners resist bringing a spouse, parent, or friend in to get the diagnosis and support that might well improve their collective lives. Depression and stress from fear and stigma of memory loss can worsen both the symptoms and the care partnership experience. Friends and family, themselves afraid of memory loss, may avoid the person experiencing it, cutting that person off from the social memory that thickened their lives and made it meaningful in the first place. It can also cause people with dementia to believe what they're being told: that their lives are meaningless.

Dementia can be frightening and disorienting for people experiencing it as well as for loved ones witnessing a person experiencing it. Negotiating systems of care can be terribly frustrating, and providing care at home can be both isolating and exhausting. The dementia experience involves grieving the changes in the person with memory loss and grieving for oneself, for one's identity that is affected by the loss of social memory—the daughter who is no longer recognized as a daughter, the spouse who is not recognized as a spouse. But the story of dementia is *also* that one's "self" persists until the end, that growth and learning are possible, that social memory remains when individual memory falters, and that relationships with a person with dementia are reciprocal. Those who do not yet have dementia do have something to learn and gain from the company of those with it.

2. Embrace the Gray

We have a tendency to see dementia in black and white. Like pregnancy, it seems, one can't be "a little bit" demented. You are or you aren't. When a person is diagnosed with mild cognitive impairment, senile dementia, or probable Alzheimer's, they might well live 15 or more years. Clearly, that time is not all a meaningless void. People can have symptom-free days, hours, minutes, or seconds. But in our current cultural moment, the fear and stigma wrapped around dementia make it seem as if diagnosis is akin to falling off a cliff. We need to follow Richard Taylor's advice. Dementia is not about half full or half empty. It's not about black or white. The experience of memory loss is gray. We need to get comfortable in the gray and keep our eyes and hearts open for moments of grace.

3. Advance the Dementia Advocacy Movement

A dementia advocacy movement, in which people with dementia and their fellow travelers fight for practical and policy changes, is just now starting to take shape. I have great hope in this movement, particularly if it is able to join forces with the extensive disability rights network. The dementia advocacy movement is roughly 20 years behind the considerable accomplishments of the various disability rights movements. There are lots of reasons for this lag. How the disability movement and aging and dementia movements have repelled each other is worthy of a dissertation (or two or three). The disability rights movement is a complex mosaic of multiple movements. It is not uncommon for various factions to disagree. The American Foundation for the Blind, for example, initially opposed the passage of the Americans with Disabilities Act on the grounds that blindness is not a disability, but a *difference*. It has also been common for groups with physical disabilities to distance themselves from those with cognitive disabilities. I asked prominent disability scholar Paul Longmore why this was so. His explanation came from personal experience. "I ride a chair," he said. "When people see the chair, they assume I am universally impaired." He spent a great deal of time overperforming on his way to a PhD to prove this wasn't the case. Although people with physical disabilities have made tremendous advances in gaining access to public places, they may hesitate to identify with and fight with and for people with cognitive disabilities.

Another reason that the dementia advocacy movement lags behind is that unlike various disability rights movement, it cannot lean heavily on economic arguments. Getting disabled people into the workforce will increase the tax base, or so the argument goes. This argument can't be used, however, with respect to retired people and those with disabilities (like late stages of Alzheimer's) severe enough to make work impossible. The catch phrase of the disability rights movement in the 1970s and '80s, "Nothing about Us without Us" fails to account for those who have great difficulty forming and expressing their thoughts.

The dementia advocacy movement has a great deal to learn from the gains and framework of the disability rights movement. "Nothing about Us without Us" would insist that people with dementia diagnoses must be part of the solution whether it is in the realm of "cure" or care. The disability rights movement learned that using tragic storylines to appeal to pity does not create lasting, positive change in the lives of people with disabilities. *No Pity,* Joseph Shapiro's chronicle of the rise of the disability rights movement, says it all. A "poster child" who raises money for a given disease is a child that is stigmatized and shamed for his or her condition. People with disabilities don't deserve pity. We all deserve to be treated with dignity. We all deserve to feel and express anger, joy, sorrow, hope, regret, and satisfaction without it being labeled a symptom.

The dementia advocacy movement should *insist on accessibility.* Ramps are increasingly being gracefully integrated into universal design. They are hardly noticeable in newer buildings. Shouldn't people with cognitive disabilities expect the same? StoryCorps and the Museum of Modern Art are both going down this path. The Meet Me at MoMA program extends MoMA's accessibility programming, which opens their collection to people with vision, hearing, and physical impairments, to people with cognitive impairments. Support for people with dementia shouldn't just come from adult day programs or assisted living or nursing home recreation activities. Cultural institutions of every size and shape should address cognitive disability in their accessibility programs and, as John Zeisel says, be part of the treatment plan for people with dementia. Can you imagine if a woman living at home with her husband felt comfortable taking him to the local art museum? or the history museum? or the botanical gardens? Imagine if they were greeted by a staff member trained in how to communicate with people with dementia rather than made to feel shame for revealing their symptoms.

The dementia advocacy movement should *take back the language of dementia.* Rather than run from the deepest stereotypes, the disability movement successfully turned them on their heads by embracing them. "Crips" and "freaks" are now terms used within the movement with pride, much in the same way that "queer" has been emptied as a pejorative. Could the worst words we can imagine to describe the experience of dementia be appropriated in a similar way? Might we reach a time when "demented" is worn on a T-shirt and reads not as an insult to the person with dementia that wears it but as an insult to the culture that shames him?

The dementia advocacy movement has some catching up to do, but it can also *teach the disability rights movement about the complexity of dependency.* The disability rights movement's focus on independence is clearly not at the core of dementia advocacy. People with dementia enter into complex relationships of care with family, friends, and paid care partners. And living in the community, alone, at home, is not always the best option for people in middle to late stages. The dementia advocacy movement can challenge the disability rights movement to more fully consider the complexity and value of *interdependency* as well as show the movement how to insist on person-centered care in nursing homes rather than simply allow them to be emptied out and shut down. I'm willing to wager that with the growing numbers of baby boomers with early diagnosis and the growing number of activists with physical disabilities now aging into cognitive disability, we'll see a joining of the disability rights and dementia advocacy movements. The field of dementia care should prepare itself now for hundreds of Richard Taylors.

4. Think Creatively and Fight for Better Options

In a survey, 355 older people revealed their fears of being diagnosed with dementia: 40 percent feared losing their insurance, 81 percent feared losing their driver's license, 50 percent feared becoming depressed, 45 percent feared becoming anxious, 38 percent feared becoming institutionalized. Compared to the fears about dementia that emerged from my own interviews (being a burden; losing control; meaninglessness; the unnaturalness of parenting your parent; being violated; becoming impoverished), these fears have downright practical solutions that should be taken up by some of our brightest minds. How can we create communities that do not rely solely on cars for transportation so that individuals who cannot drive can easily, and with some spontaneity, get where they need to go (without waiting half the day and feeling their blood boil)? How can we make sure that cognitive impairment does not preclude people from getting the health care they deserve? Can we imagine better options to the current nursing home, which is oriented to the needs of the institution overall rather the well-being of individual residents? These are changes that could improve the lives of many, many people, not just those with dementia.

5. Think and Act in Coalition

To reduce stigma and improve the quality of life for people living with dementia, we need to act in coalition. This is tricky. Because the stigma of dementia is so strong, potential coalition partners might prefer to keep their distance. But just as I am suggesting that we need to see the self and memory as relational, we also need to acknowledge that dementia advocates will never make meaningful change on their own. Dementia advocates need to reach out to groups that share their challenges and can benefit from their victories. We need to use our energies to stand by our partners as well. As Peter Whitehouse points out, environmental toxins are damaging the cognitive health of everyone, and kids with lead poisoning will be the next generation of adults with dementia. Farm subsidies provide incentives for producing high-fat, corn-fed cattle and high-fructose corn syrup, which contribute to obesity, heart disease, and diabetes. Research now tells us that heart health is closely linked to brain health. Might the American Heart Association be a partner in dementia advocacy? Might people in early-stage dementia fight farm subsidies? We need to think creatively about who might share a mission to improve the quality of life among people with cognitive disabilities, build relationships, and get savvy about how to make change. I can imagine an ACT UP–style action in which people of a range of ages and disabilities along with staff, families, and friends link arms and surround a nursing home, all wearing T-shirts that say "Demented and Proud!"

6. Value Listening, Silence, and the Present Moment

The StoryCorps project invites us to listen as an act of love. David Greenberger lobs questions that dare people to respond. And then he listens. TimeSlips creates a setting in which facilitators listen to and echo the words of people with dementia, making sure to get the pitch, tone, and emotional intent just right as they weave all the answers into story. Songwriting Works does the same but builds the responses into song. All the programs that I profile in part 3 find a way to suspend Western culture's high-speed churning of the future into the past. They invite us into the present moment, deep listening, and occasional silence—a place that feels increasingly foreign in our multitasking culture of distraction. Gaining comfort in the present moment can remind us of the mysteries of being alive. I'm not good at writing about this. I start to giggle, or worse, when I get into spiritual territory. There are many people who do it eloquently, particularly people who study Buddhism. All I can say is that spending time with people who have dementia has made me a more patient parent, friend, daughter, sister, and wife. It's made me notice and be endlessly thankful for things like the horizon of Lake Michigan, gray storm clouds, three or four well-chosen notes on a cello, and breathing.

7. Understand That Memory Is More Than Individual Property

Every model of memory that I've found in psychology books neatly shows various types of memories and how an *individual* processes them. These models are helpful, memory being as complex as it is. But all these drawings should all have an asterisk: *Note: this model does not exist outside of the laboratory. Memory is social. But this fact doesn't lend itself to neat diagrams. The field of memory studies, which explores the collective and social nature of memory, is growing. In 1998, Jeffrey Olick called the field "centerless." The two books Olick has written since provide it with a bit more solid footing. In January 2008, Sage Publications came out with the first issue of *Memory Studies,* a journal drawing from disciplines such as philosophy, psychology, history, sociology, and anthropology. Perhaps one of these scholars will come up with a diagram that neatly shows the various kinds of memory and how we process them, not as individuals in a lab setting, but as real people, in real relationships with friends, family, work, and communities at large.

There are two basic definitions of memory. The first refers to our traditional sense of memory, of bringing the past into the present. The second refers to forming community. "Remember me to your parents," we might say to a friend. "Remember me to your husband." We human creatures never lose our need or capacity for this type of memory—of making one's self a member of a community—even when we are in the depths of dementia.

We must remember that memory is social, that the "self" is relational. To forget this is to ignore one of our best "cures" for memory loss—creating a net of social memory around a person whose individual control of memory is compromised. This doesn't mean that we should *visit* people more. This means that people with memory loss need to be reknit into the fabric of our lives. The members of a nursing home staff shouldn't think of a spouse or a son or a daughter or a friend as a *visitor.* They should think of them as part of their *community.*

8. Healing Is Bigger Than Memory

Some amazing activists, artists, and therapists out there are using their skills to heal individuals and communities. These can be people haunted by single traumatic events (9/11, Oklahoma City, school shootings) or by the multitude of daily traumas that war, poverty, or neglect can breed. "Memory" is commonly a theme in the work of healing. Activists, artists, or therapists gather and share the stories and voices of survivors of all kinds in an effort to knit past with present and, it is to be hoped, envision and step toward a transformed future. But memory is not the only road to healing. People with memory loss, even those in the late stages, can heal too. Shared communication of any kind, be it through music, movement, visual art, poetry, or storytelling, can bring people suffering from loneliness and isolation into community. Perhaps simply shifting the language of healing so that it leans less on *memory* and more on something like *shared visions* will help reduce the pressure put on memory to be the locus of all hope for healing.

9. Assert the Value of Forgetting

Prompted by a party game after a few glasses of wine, Umberto Eco came up with an idea for a conference paper: it is impossible to have an "art of forgetting." According to Eco's paper, called playfully "An *Ars Oblivionalis?* Forget It," all signs produce presences, not absences, and you can't create a sign for something you want to disappear. But if we can't have an "art of forgetting," we *can* remember the value of forgetting and of those who forget. Forgetting can be a good and healthy thing. Letting names, numbers, places fall through our netting enables us to focus on other, possibly more important things. Heiner Müller forcefully champions cultural memory when he writes, "There is no revolution without a memory." And clearly, large-scale, cultural forgetting makes it possible for us to repeat horrors of our past, such as genocide. But on an individual scale, a certain amount of forgetting also enables us to see the forest, not just thousands of individual trees with millions of individual needles. Forgetting makes us human.

10. Insist That It Is Normal for Young People to Care about Aging

Actress Sarah Polley was not strange for making her directorial debut, *Away from Her,* on the topic of Alzheimer's disease. Stefan Merrill Block was not strange for taking early-onset Alzheimer's as the subject of his superb debut novel, *The Story of Forgetting.* Memory loss, dying, and aging itself put us directly in touch with what it means to be human, to love, to be faithful, to live a meaningful life. Great philosophers and artists since the beginning of time have tackled these issues. Who *wouldn't* want to think about that? All the young people who harbor interest in working with older adults should stop worrying whether people will think they are strange. I find it much odder to actively avoid thinking about aging or being with older people and, in doing so, deliberately detach oneself from some of the greatest mysteries of life.

11. Open Avenues for Meaning-Making

According to terror management theory, anything that reminds us of death makes us anxious and we avoid it, whether it is a dangerous situation or a person with dementia. For some people, normal, age-related memory gaffs are their first palpable taste of mortality. Their panic is, in part, fear of this unwanted reminder of death and disability. But at the end of the day, I don't think death is at the root of our fears of memory loss. The losses in the experience of dementia are thick and recurring. I believe our fear of memory loss is rooted in a fear that these losses will overwhelm us and those close to us and drain all meaning from the relationships and accomplishments we've spent years of physical and emotional labor to build. We fear that we will sit, or watch our loved ones sit, in a meaningless void for years until the body catches up with the brain, and we finally die.

Dr. Christine Kovach, a colleague at the University of Wisconsin–Milwaukee, works almost exclusively with people who have late-stage dementia. Based on her extensive research, she came up with a way for nursing staff to respond to what are called "problem behaviors" in nursing homes, like screaming, hitting, or basically doing the wrong thing at the wrong time in the wrong place. When people with late-stage dementia exhibit a "problem behavior," Kovach asks the staff to consider what they might be trying to communicate. Are they in pain? Part of her care plan asks the staff to determine if people in late stages are getting at least 10 minutes of "meaningful human interaction" per day. Meaningful human interaction can be a hand massage or simply someone sitting and talking to them. It is heartbreaking to think that we'd need Dr. Kovach's assessment guidelines. It is heartbreaking to know that just 10 minutes can make such a big difference. And it's even more heartbreaking to know that there are many, many people with dementia who go without those 10 minutes, whether they live at home or in facilities.

The arts provide a way to open those avenues for meaning-making between people who cannot communicate through traditional, rational language. Music and songwriting, dance, nonlinear storytelling, poetry, open conversation, painting, sculpting, responding to art: all of these give us ways to connect with each other, express who we are and what we believe. They can help put meaning back into what we fear are meaningless lives.

You don't need to be a certified therapist to create moments of meaningful engagement. As Liz Lerman said so eloquently, there is a busy highway between the extremes of the arts. On the one end are the elite arts, like the ballet and the opera that we watch with amazement. On the other end are the therapists who, in some situations, really are the only people qualified to help a patient. But on the busy highway between these two extremes, there are Katie Williams and the Good Steppers of Luther Manor. There are the volunteer artists reading and writing poetry at adult day centers. There is you. There is me.

Unfortunately, I can't cite statistics about the power of the arts that policy makers will trust enough to put money behind getting arts training and programs into every care setting for people with dementia. There are no large-scale, double-blind, controlled studies of programs that open meaning-making between care partners and people with dementia. Thus far, major research dollars have bypassed these nonpharmacological treatments. I understand the urge to put the vast majority of research dollars into bench science. We want a pill, and we want a pill fast. But a large-scale study with relatively healthy older adults tells us that being involved in art making reduces depression and the number of doctor visits and improves self-esteem, a sense of being socially supported, all while stabilizing general health. Do we think that the impact on people with cognitive disabilities will be so radically different? Small-scale studies tell us that dance reduces cognitive disability. Small-scale studies tell us that visual arts programs improve mood and quality of life for people with dementia. And that storytelling increases the quality and quantity of interactions between staff and residents with dementia in nursing homes. We need research that convinces policy makers that training care partners to foster meaningful moments with people with dementia might work better than pills, and without side effects. Meaning-making might even work to reduce stigma and fear, something a pill can never do.

12. Don't Be Afraid of Reducing Fear

What exactly would *happen* if we reduced stigma and fear? After talking with hundreds of people who work in the field of dementia care, I've come to believe that we're *afraid* to reduce the fear of dementia. We think that reducing fear will mean a sudden plunge in the amount of research dollars that come from private donors and the NIH alike. We think it would mean that the term "Alzheimer's," that strange-sounding German word that ill fits our tongues (Al-timer's? old-timers?) will fade out of use just as the Alzheimer's Association, which provides so many valuable services, struggles to get its name and services out to every American household that needs them. We fear that people will stop blaming a "disease" and will blame the person with dementia for acting funny ("If he loved me, he wouldn't forget these things"). Stigma and fear are evolutionary impulses, some theories would have us believe; they help us identify people not to marry, people that might be harmful to us. We think we *need* the stigma and fear of dementia.

Perhaps if we can imagine the *benefits* of reducing stigma and fear, it will give us courage to take the plunge. What might happen if we reduced the fear and stigma of dementia?

More people might get diagnosed.

More people might plan ahead, with long-term care insurance; more people might have family discussions about what to do if they should experience dementia.

More people might learn about and use services that enable them to stay at home, if that is their choice.

More people might spend more time with more friends who live in nursing homes.

If more people spent time in nursing homes, there might be less tolerance for poor-quality care and poor quality of life.

Less stigma and fear might reduce stress for people with dementia, which might improve cognition.

Friends and family might be more involved and supportive of care partners and people with dementia, reducing social isolation.

More social support might mean less stress for care partners, improving their health.

Less stigma and fear might give us better attitudes about aging—and longer lives (we could win back our 7.5 years).

More people might go into the field of dementia care, which could lead to innovations in all areas, from housing to care services.

More options for care might mean less stress for working adults managing care for their parents.

Less stress for working adults might mean greater productivity in the workplace.

Cultural institutions might acknowledge people with cognitive disabilities as valued members of the community they serve.

People with dementia and their care partners might feel more comfortable visiting cultural institutions that welcome them, again reducing stress and challenging and growing their cognitive skills.

Maybe we would take lifelong learning (not just computerized cognitive exercises) a little more seriously.

Maybe dementia advocates would find kinship with other groups advocating for lifelong cognitive and physical health and forge effective coalitions.

Maybe we would actually develop a long-term care policy in the United States.

Maybe we would have more people who have 10 minutes of meaningful human interaction per day.

Maybe we would reduce "problem behaviors."

Maybe we would learn something about the meaning of life from people living intensely in the present, a place those without cognitive disability rarely get to experience.

Maybe we would grow as human beings by expanding our capacity for compassion.

One of the quiet prides I have of my family is my father's vocabulary. Thomas John Basting was the only child of Alice Koehn and Abe Basting. Abe and Alice lived in a little bungalow that Alice's father built on the South Side of Milwaukee, where Alice's family experienced and survived the Depression. Alice worked as an assistant to a lawyer and Abe sold shoes. My father vividly remembers the day his mother walked him to the bursar's office at Marquette University and wrote a tuition check for $500. He had no earthly idea where she came up with that money. A college education was Abe and Alice's dream for their only child. It would give him keys to the world of the people they typed letters for and fitted for fancy shoes. But sometimes I think my father's access to that other world came more from his masterful command of language than from his college education. Even now, when a little-used,

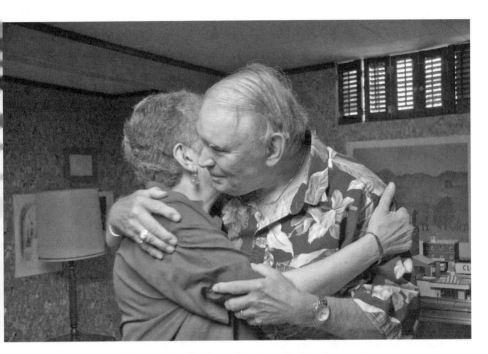

Roger and Rocille McConnell. Photo by www.jimherrington.com.

strange-sounding, and perfect word slips from my lips into conversation, I know it came from him. If and when I face dementia and lose my facility with time and language, I will not only struggle to express myself to others (and myself), I will lose my father as well. And that scares me.

If dementia comes to me, there will be losses, and possibly other, sometimes frightening, symptoms related to dementia. But, I hope, if and when I start to show symptoms of dementia, there will also be a chance for me to have a meaningful life from beginning to end. I hope that it will be possible for the story of who I am to continue as something more than a simple tragedy. That is the case for Roger and Rocille, who, in spite of their considerable fears, move through Roger's dementia with the expectation that their friends and family will open themselves to learning about the condition and that their health professionals will treat them with dignity. Dementia hasn't stopped them from being actively engaged in their community or from exploring the world. They added Sicily to the map of their world travels in 2007. In 2008, they visited the pyramids. Roger and Rocille don't stop at fear. Roger and Rocille are so much more than dementia. Aren't we all?

QUESTION: If you had magic and could change one thing about Alzheimer's (without curing it) what would it be?

DEBBIE: I would fix the fear. As a nurse and caregiver, I feel the most helpless when I'm caring for someone with Alzheimer's disease and they are fearful and I'm not able to alleviate the fear. If I had a magic wand, I would remove the fear factor. Not just the fear of the early diagnosis of where they are headed, but when the disease advances, where am I? Why am I here? To alleviate that fear would be huge.

Appendix A
Program Description and Contact Information

Alzheimer's Association
The Alzheimer's Association is the leading voluntary health organization in Alzheimer's care, support, and research; it has a national office and regional chapters across the United States.
President and CEO: Harry Johns
www.alz.org
National help line: 800-272-3900

ArtCare
ArtCare, run by Luther Manor Adult Day Services in Milwaukee began in 1994 and offers annual artist residencies in music, dance, storytelling, and a variety of visual arts. Artists in residence teach the staff how to continue the programs after their residencies are over. All residencies culminate in a public celebration of the work.
Director: Beth Meyer Arnold
www.luthermanor.org
Contact: 414-464-3888
Resources:
    ArtCare manual (www.aging.uwm.edu)

Artists for Alzheimer's (ARTZ)
Based at Hearthstone Alzheimer's Care and founded by John Zeisel in 2001, ARTZ is a nonprofit, membership-based organization that trains artist volunteers to work with people with dementia in facility-based care settings and that manages their volunteer activity. Hearthstone also offers consulting services on designing programs and facilities for people with dementia.
Directors: John Zeisel and Sean Caulfield
www.thehearth.org/artistsforalzheimers.htm
Contact: 781-844-4671 or Caulfield@TheHearth.org
Resources:
    T-shirts for sale to support ARTZ

Arts for the Aging (AFTA)

Founded in 1988 by sculptor Lolo Sarnoff, AFTA has a faculty of 18 artists who provide (for free) up to 33 programs a year to partnering organizations based in the metropolitan Washington, D.C., area. AFTA offers trainings and is focused on underserved seniors.

Executive director: Janine Tursini
Program director: Diana Cirone
www.aftaarts.org
Contact: 301-718-4990 or info@aftaarts.org

Center for Elders and Youth in the Arts (CEYA)

CEYA provides specialized visual and performing arts programming, much done in collaboration with youth groups, tailored to the San Francisco Bay–area older adult population. Since 1996, CEYA has served thousands of elders and hundreds of youth.

Artistic director: Jeff Chapline
http://ceya.ioaging.org
Contact: 415-447-1989, ext. 534, or ceya@ioaging.org

DanceWorks

DanceWorks teaching artists work in adult day settings in Milwaukee offering dance workshops and intergenerational multiarts programs (IMAP).

Executive director: Deborah Farris
www.danceworksmke.org
Contact: 414-277-8480

Duplex Planet

Unconventional interviews with older adults conducted by founder David Greenberger are transformed into various works of art.

www.duplexplanet.com
Contact: info@duplexplanet.com
Resources:
    back issues of *Duplex Planet* journals
    CDs
    books

Elders Share the Arts (ESTA)

Founded by Susan Perlstein in 1979, ESTA offers a range of programs, including the Legacy Works program, which uses visual arts to tell stories.

Executive director: Carolyn Zablotny
Program director: Marsha Gildin
www.elderssharethearts.org

Contact: 718-398-3870
Resources:

*A Stage for Memory: A Guide to the Living History Theater Program of
Elders Share the Arts*

The Arts and Dementia Care: A Resource Guide

Legacy Works: Visual Art and Reminiscence for Older Adults

*Generating Community: Intergenerational Partnerships through the
Expressive Arts*

Other books, manuals, and videos

The Intergenerational School

The Intergenerational School is a nationally recognized, Cleveland-based K–8
charter school whose mission is to foster an educational community of excellence that provides experiences and skills for lifelong learning and spirited citizenship for learners of all ages.

www.tisonline.org

Contact: 216-721-0120 or info@tisonline.org

Kairos Dance Theatre

A Minneapolis-based intergenerational dance company, Kairos was founded
by Maria Genné in 1991 and began its programs for people with memory loss
in 2001. It now offers training and runs dance programs at multiple sites
every year.

Artistic director: Maria Genné

www.kairosdance.org

Contact: info@kairosdance.org

Liz Lerman Dance Exchange

Founded in 1976 by Liz Lerman, Dance Exchange has created more than 50
dance/theater works. It has held thousands of performances and sponsored
many community exchanges. Its free, online toolbox shares valuable exercises
designed to encourage group participation and creative expression.

Producing artistic director: Peter DiMuro

www.danceexchange.org

Contact: mail@danceexchange.org

Memories in the Making

Memories in the Making, founded by Selly Jenny in 1986, is a failure-free art
program designed to encourage self-expression by people with dementia. The
program originally focused on watercolor painting, but individual Alzheimer's
Association chapters have adapted/expanded Memories in the Making as it
has spread across the country. See, for example, the Cincinnati chapter, the

Greater Wisconsin chapter, the southeastern Wisconsin chapter, the heartland chapter, and the Denver chapter.
Managed by the Orange County chapter of the Alzheimer's Association
National trainer: La Doris "Sam" Heinly
www.alz.org/oc/in_my_community_10849.asp
Contact: 949-757-3719 (Orange County program)
Resources:
> *Memories in the Making Training Manual* and DVD
> *I'm Still Here,* by Sam Heinly, featuring paintings of people with dementia

Memory Bridge
Memory Bridge is a curriculum to teach middle and senior high school students about memory and identity through partnerships with people with dementia. The Memory Bridge curriculum is available for purchase, and comes with training and support. *There Is a Bridge* is a documentary film produced by Memory Bridge founder Michael Verde in 2007 and distributed by American Public Media.
President: Michael Verde
www.memorybridge.org
Contact: Athena Rebapis, outreach coordinator, arebapis@Mbeducation.net

Museum of Modern Art
Education and Access for Visitors with Disabilities and Special Needs
The museum's Meet Me at MoMA Program offers tours for people with dementia and their caregivers on a day when the museum is closed to the public. This program is free but requires registration.
www.moma.org/education/moma_access.html
Contact: 212-408-6347 or 212-247-230 (TTY) or
Alzheimersproject@moma.org
Resources:
> *MoMA Alzheimer's Project Guide for Museums*

National Center for Creative Aging (NCCA)
Founded in 2001, NCCA is a membership organization "dedicated to fostering an understanding of the vital relationship between creative expression and healthy aging and to developing programs that build on this understanding."
Executive director: Gay Hanna
www.creativeaging.org
Contact: 202-895-9456 or info@creativeaging.org

Resources:
  arts and aging national resource directory
  NCCA newsletter
  Creativity Matters: The Arts and Aging Tool Kit

Neighbors Growing Together

Neighbors Growing Together is a program at Virginia Tech whose mission is "to improve the lives of people across the lifespan through intergenerational collaboration involving teaching, research, and outreach." www.intergenerational.clahs.vt.edu/neighbors/index.html
Contact: 540-231-5434 or sjarrot@vt.edu

Next Stage Dance Theater (NSDT)

Based in Seattle and cofounded by Dominique Gabella and Bridget Thompson in 1999, NSDT initiated its Unleashed Memories program for people with dementia in 2005 and now runs it at two to three sites per year.
Artistic director: Dominique Gabella
www.nextstagedance.org
Contact: 206-633-0812, ext. 3, or info@nextstagedance.org

Songwriting Works

An internationally recognized creative organization founded in 1990 by Judith-Kate Friedman that promotes health through the power of songwriting and performance, Songwriting Works offers training and sponsors residencies in facilities across the country.
Director: Judith-Kate Friedman
www.songwritingworks.org
Contact: 360-385-1160 or info@songwritingworks.org
Resources:
  CDs
  An Especially Wonderful Affair
  prints of articles by Friedman
  training materials forthcoming

St. Ann Center for Intergenerational Care

St. Ann Center for Intergenerational Care is a Milwaukee-based intergenerational day-care center that strives to prevent premature institutionalization of elderly people and persons with disabilities. Photographer Wing Young Huie photographed extensively at St. Ann's Good Shepherd House, an adult day program for people with dementia.
www.stanncenter.org
Contact: 414-977-5000 (main office)

StoryCorps

StoryCorps, founded by David Isay in 2003, is a national oral history project whose mission is to honor and celebrate one another's lives through listening. The Memory Loss Initiative of StoryCorps began in 2006.
Executive director: David Isay
Director of StoryCorps: Donna Galeno
Senior outreach coordinator, Memory Loss Initiative: Dina Zempsky
www.storycorps.net
Contact: 646-723-7027 (general questions); 800-850-4406 (reservations)
Resources:
> *Listening Is an Act of Love* (a book that shares the history and stories of the StoryCorps project)

Talk Back Move Forward: 100 Years of Alzheimer's Disease

Talk Back Move Forward is an 8-minute video based on photographs of and interviews with people with dementia, medical researchers, and family and professional caregivers.
Producer and director: Anne Basting
Available for free download at www.aging.uwm.edu

TimeSlips

A group storytelling process founded by Anne Basting that encourages people to imagine rather than remember. There are currently 12 TimeSlips training bases across the country. TimeSlips offers consulting and training on using creative expression in person-centered dementia care.
Director: Anne Basting
www.timeslips.org
Contact: info@timeslips.org
Resources:
> TimeSlips training manual (50 pages)
> TimeSlips DVD (12 minutes)
> images for storytelling sessions

To Whom I May Concern

Founded by Maureen Matthews (PhD), *To Whom I May Concern* is a play and a process for weaving together a play from the words of people with dementia.
www.towhomimayconcern.org
Contact: info@towhomimayconcern.org

United Community Center (UCC)

The Milwaukee-based UCC provides programs to the Hispanic community and residents in Near South Side of all ages in the areas of education, cultural arts, recreation, community development, and health and human services. UCC helps people achieve their potential by focusing on cultural heritage as a means of strengthening personal development. Photographer Wing Young Huie worked extensively at UCC's adult day center.

Adult day center coordinator: Nelva Olin

www.unitedcc.org

Contact: 414-384-3100 (main office); 414-384-3100, ext. 4709 (adult day center)

Wing Young Huie

Wing Young Huie is a nationally recognized documentary photographer who began to photograph people with memory loss in 2006 as part of his residency in applied art at the University of Wisconsin–Milwaukee's Center on Age and Community.

www.wingyounghuie.com

Contact: info@wingyounghuie.com

Appendix B
Recipes from Chapter 1

Gülgün Kayim's Shepherd's Pie

> 2 tablespoons canola oil
> 1 pound or so ground meat
> 1 medium onion, chopped
> 1 small carrot
> $\frac{1}{4}$ cup peas
> 1 stalk celery
> 2–3 tablespoons Marmite (English brown goop)
> 1 bay leaf
> 2–3 teaspoons oregano
> $\frac{1}{4}$ cup water or chicken or beef stock
> salt and pepper to taste

For the mashed topping:

> 3 cups water
> 5–6 medium potatoes
> $\frac{1}{4}$ cup plus 2 tablespoons milk (reserve 2 tablespoons for topping)
> 4–5 tablespoons butter
> salt and pepper to taste

Preheat oven to 350 degrees. Fill large pot with water and put on to boil. Peel and chop potatoes; add to water when boiling. In a large pan, fry onion in oil until soft. Add ground meat and brown. Add carrots, celery, oregano, salt, pepper, Marmite; stir and cook for 5 minutes. Add liquid and bay leaf, and simmer for 10 minutes. Add peas, cook for 5 minutes, remove from heat, and pour filling into a 9-inch square Pyrex baking pan. Check potatoes for doneness; remove and mash when ready, adding butter, milk, salt, and pepper. Spread evenly over the ground meat mixture, brush with a little milk, and put into center of oven. Bake for 45 minutes, or until the mashed topping is brown. Serve hot from the oven with a green salad.

Thom Sobota's Cheesecake

Crust:

> 1 stick butter
> 10 graham crackers
> $\frac{1}{2}$ cup sugar

Pulse melted butter, grahams, and sugar in a food processor until moist and crushed. Spoon into a springform pan and pat down.

Cake:

> 2 eggs
> 2 8-ounce packages cream cheese, softened
> $\frac{1}{2}$ cup sugar
> 1 teaspoon vanilla

Blend until smooth and pour on top of the crust in the springform pan.
Bake at 375 degrees for 20 minutes. You should see the edges of the cake beginning to crack. Let cool for 15 minutes.

Topping:

> 16 ounces sour cream (low fat is okay)
> $\frac{1}{4}$ cup sugar
> 1 tablespoon vanilla

Mix thoroughly and spread on top of cooled cheesecake. Bake at 425 degrees for 5 minutes.
   Cool in refrigerator for at least 3 hours before serving.

Appendix C
Images and Stories of Dementia

Novels

Bernlef, J. Trans. Adrienne Dixon. *Out of Mind.* London: Faber and Faber, 1988.

Block, Stefan Merrill. *The Story of Forgetting.* New York: Random House, 2008.

Franzen, Jonathan. *The Corrections.* New York: Farrar, Straus and Giroux, 2001.

Genova, Lisa. *Still Alice.* iUniverse, 2007.

Ignatieff, Michael. *Scar Tissue.* New York: Farrar, Straus and Giroux, 1994.

Plays

Carson, Jo. *Daytrips.* New York: Dramatist's Play Service, 1998.

Congdon, Constance. *Tales of the Lost Formicans.* New York: Broadway Play Publishing, 1990.

Foote, Horton. *The Last of the Thorntons.* New York: Dramatist's Play Service, 2002.

Lonergan, Kenneth. *The Waverly Gallery.* New York: Grove Press, 2000.

Mighton, John. *Half Life.* Toronto: Playwrights Canada Press, 2006.

Vradenburg, Trish. *Surviving Grace.* New York: Broadway Play Publishing, 2003.

Memoirs and Autobiographies

Bayley, John. *Elegy for Iris.* New York: St. Martin's Press, 1999.

Bryden, Christine. *Dancing with Dementia: My Story of Living Positively with Dementia.* London: Jessica Kingsley Publishers, 2005.

Davidson, Ann. *Alzheimer's, a Love Story: One Year in My Husband's Journey.* New York: Carol Publishing, 1997.

———. *A Curious Kind of Widow: Loving a Man with Advanced Alzheimer's.* McKinleyville, CA: Daniel and Daniel, 2006.

Davis, Robert. *My Journey into Alzheimer's Disease.* Wheaton, IL: Tyndale House Publishers, 1989.

DeBaggio, Thomas. *Losing My Mind: An Intimate Look at Life with Alzheimer's.* New York: Free Press, 2002.

————. *When It Gets Dark: An Enlightened Reflection on Life with Alzheimer's.* New York: Free Press, 2003.

Fuchs, Elinor. *Making an Exit: A Mother-Daughter Drama with Machine Tools, Alzheimer's, and Laughter.* New York: Metropolitan Books, 2005.

Henderson, Cary. *Partial View: An Alzheimer's Journal.* Dallas, TX: Southern Methodist University Press, 1998.

Lee, Jeanne. *Just Love Me.* West Lafayette, IN: Purdue University Press, 2003.

McGowin, Diana Friel. *Living in the Labyrinth.* New York: Delacorte Press, 1993.

Miller, Sue. *The Story of My Father: A Memoir.* New York: Knopf, 2003.

Mobley, Tracy. *Young Hope: The Broken Road.* Parker, CO: Outskirts Press, 2007.

Rose, Larry. *Larry's Way: Another Look at Alzheimer's from the Inside.* Lincoln, NE: iUniverse, 2003.

————. *Show Me the Way to Go Home.* Forest Knolls, CA: Elder Books, 1995.

Schneider, Charles. *Don't Bury Me . . . It Ain't Over Yet.* Milton Keynes, UK: AuthorHouse, 2006.

Taylor, Richard. *Alzheimer's from the Inside Out.* Baltimore: Health Professions Press, 2007.

Other Nonfiction

Greenberger, David. *Duplex Planet: Everybody's Asking Who I Was.* Boston: Faber and Faber, 1994.

Greenblat, Cathy Stein. *Alive with Alzheimer's.* Chicago: University of Chicago Press, 2004.

Peterson, Betsy. *Voices of Alzheimer's: Courage, Humor, Hope, and Love in the Face of Dementia.* Cambridge, MA: Da Capo Press, 2004.

Shenk, David. *The Forgetting: Alzheimer's, Portrait of an Epidemic.* New York: Doubleday, 2001.

Snyder, Lisa. *Speaking Our Minds: Personal Reflections from Individuals with Alzheimer's.* New York: W. H. Freeman, 1999.

Strauss Smoller, Esther. *I Can't Remember: Family Stories of Alzheimer's Disease.* Philadelphia: Temple University Press, 1997.

Television/Film

Aurora Borealis. Written by Brent Boyd and directed by James Burke, 2005.
Away from Her. Written and directed by Sarah Polley, adapted from a short story by Alice Munro, 2006.
Complaints of a Dutiful Daughter. Documentary by Deborah Hoffman, 1995.
Diminished Capacity. Written by Sherwood Kiraly and directed by Terry Kinney, 2008.
Do Not Go Gently. Documentary by Melissa Godoy and Eileen Littig, 2007.
Do You Remember Love? Written by Vickie Patik and directed by Jeff Bleckner, 1985.
Iris. Written and directed by Richard Eyre, adapted from a book by John Bayley, 2001.
Memory for Max, Clare, Ida and Company. Documentary by Alan King, 2005.
Pop. Documentary by Joel Meyerowitz, 1999.
The Good Life. Written and directed by Stephen Berra, 2007.
The Savages. Written and directed by Tamara Jenkins, 2007.
There Is a Bridge. Documentary by Michael Verde, 2007.

Web-based

www.aboutalz.org. *A Quick Look at Alzheimer's: Four "Pocket" Films to Increase Understanding of a 21st Century Epidemic,* produced and directed by David Shenk.
www.alz.org. National Alzheimer's Association site, which includes an online forum for people with dementia.
www.alzsh.net. Alzheimer's Spoken Here, a resource for people carrying diagnoses similar to Alzheimer's disease.
www.dasninternational.org. Dementia Advocacy and Support Network International.
www.dementiausa.com. Online support for people with dementia.
www.duplexplanet.com. David Greenberger's Duplex Planet.
www.storycorps.net. The national StoryCorps project, including the Memory Loss Initiative.

Appendix D
Timeline of Stories and Events in the Recent History of Dementia

1980
"Dear Abby" column features a letter about Alzheimer's disease and generates 30,000 responses.

The Senate Subcommittee on Aging conducts hearings on the impact of Alzheimer's disease on the nation's elderly.

The National Institute on Aging's *Age Page* publishes "Senility: Myth or Madness?"

1981
The 36-Hour Day, by Nancy Mace and Peter Rabins, is published.

Charles Leroux writes a column titled "A Silent Epidemic" for the *Chicago Tribune.*

The Myth of Senility: The Truth about the Brain and Aging, by Robin Marantz Henig, is published.

1982
The first public service announcement about Alzheimer's, with Jack Lemmon, airs.

President Ronald Reagan signs a proclamation designating the fourth week in November National Alzheimer's Disease Awareness Week.

1983
The House Select Committee on Aging holds hearings on senility and stereotyping.

The Senate Subcommittee on Aging holds hearings on living with Alzheimer's.

1984
Newsweek reports on Alzheimer's, featuring "The Agony of Alzheimer's Disease" on its cover and publishing "A Slow Death of the Mind" by Matt Clark (December).

1985

"Alzheimer's Disease," by Richard J. Wurtman, is published in *Scientific American* (January).

Patti LuPone records "It's a Long Goodbye" for the Alzheimer's Disease and Related Disorders Association.

The Alzheimer's Disease and Related Disorders Association produces a documentary entitled "Caring."

Do You Remember Love? airs on CBS, starring Joanne Woodward as a poet and college instructor with Alzheimer's (May).

1986

The House Select Committee on Aging holds hearings on the burdens of Alzheimer's disease for victims and their families.

The Loss of Self: A Family Resource for the Care of Alzheimer's Disease and Related Disorders, by Donna Cohen and Carl Eisdorfer, is published.

1987

Oprah Winfrey features Alzheimer's disease on her show.

1988

The Alzheimer's Disease and Related Disorders Association airs a public service announcement titled "Stand by You," and the organization changes its name to the Alzheimer's Association.

Willard Scott is named national spokesperson for the Alzheimer's Association.

Understanding Alzheimer's Disease, edited by Miriam Aronson, is published.

Out of Mind, a novel by J. Bernlef, is published.

1989

A *Journal of the American Medical Association* article states that four million Americans have Alzheimer's disease.

1990

A public service announcement about the statistic that four million Americans suffer from Alzheimer's disease airs with Walter Cronkite.

The Living Death, a "supermarket paperback," is published by the National Foundation for Medical Research.

Janet Adkins is Jack Kevorkian's first "client." The *New York Times* ("Her Mind Was Everything, Dead Woman's Husband Says" by Timothy Eagan [June 6]) and *Time* magazine cover the story.

1991
"Alzheimer's: Is There Hope?" appears as a cover story in *U.S. News and World Report* (August).
HBO special, *Losing It All,* airs (October).

1993
Cognex, a drug to treat Alzheimer's, is approved.
The Alzheimer's Association's "Warning Signs" awareness campaign draws a huge response.
As the World Turns character Mac learns he has Alzheimer's disease.
Living in the Labyrinth, by Diana Friel McGowin, is published.

1994
Reagan announces he has Alzheimer's disease.
Scar Tissue, a novel by Michael Ignatieff, is published.
Duplex Planet: Everybody's Asking Who I Was, by David Greenberger, is published.
ER airs two episodes with Rosemary Clooney playing a singing Alzheimer's patient (September and December).

1995
The Alzheimer's Association launches its first Web site.
Nancy Reagan's public service announcement about Alzheimer's airs.
Beverly Hills 90210 episode with Milton Berle playing Saul Howard, a character with Alzheimer's disease, airs (January).

1996
Aricept is approved to treat Alzheimer's.
USA Network's *Road to Galveston,* starring Tess Harper, about widow who provides care for three women with Alzheimer's disease, airs (January).
The Notebook, by Nicholas Sparks, is published.

1997
An excerpt from Joel Meyerowitz's documentary *Pop* ("Defying Sickness") airs on WBEZ Chicago's *This American Life* (August).
Alzheimer's, a Love Story: One Year in My Husband's Journey, by Ann Davidson, is published.

1998
The Alzheimer's Association's women and Alzheimer's disease campaign ad with Patti LaBelle airs on television and radio.

David Hyde Pierce testifies before Congress on the projection of 14 million baby boomers developing Alzheimer's disease.

A Partial View: An Alzheimer's Journal, by Cary Henderson, is published.

1999

Elegy for Iris, by John Bayley, is published. Murdoch dies.

Thomas DeBaggio is on NPR for the first time (December).

Speaking Our Minds: Personal Expressions from Individuals with Alzheimer's, edited by Lisa Snyder, is published.

PBS's *Frontline* airs Joel Meyerowitz's documentary *Pop* (June).

2000

The Alzheimer's Association's public service announcement with Rita Hayworth airs.

Newsweek and *Time* feature cover articles on Alzheimer's disease (January and July).

Excelon, a new Alzheimer's drug, is approved.

Thomas DeBaggio gives updates on NPR's *All Things Considered* (March, July, and November).

The Waverly Gallery, by Kenneth Lonergan, is produced at Promenade in New York City.

The Waverly Gallery is published.

"The New Science of Alzheimer's," by Madeleine Nash, is published in *Time* (July).

Hard to Forget: An Alzheimer's Story, by Charles Pierce, is published.

Decoding Darkness: The Search for the Genetic Causes of Alzheimer's Disease, by Rudolph Tanzi and Ann Parson, is published.

2001

The drug Razadyne is approved to treat Alzheimer's.

The film *Iris* is released (December).

The Forgetting: Alzheimer's, Portrait of an Epidemic, by David Shenk, is published.

The Corrections, a novel by Jonathan Franzen, is published.

"The Nun Study," by Michael Lemonick and Alice Park, is published in *Time* (May).

2002

National Alzheimer's Disease Awareness Month is declared.

The Alzheimer's Association's public service announcement "Faces of Alzheimer's," with David Hyde Pierce, airs.

Losing My Mind, a memoir by Thomas DeBaggio, is published.

2003

The drug Namenda is approved.

The Alzheimer's Association airs "Dear Abby" and "Spanish Happy Birthday" public service announcements.

When It Gets Dark, by Thomas DeBaggio, is published.

Story of My Father: A Memoir, by Sue Miller, is published.

2004

The Forgetting appears on PBS (January). One thousand house parties are held during its airing.

Ronald Reagan dies; the Alzheimer's Association is named one of three official memorial charities.

The Alzheimer's Association launches its "Maintain Your Brain" campaign and creates a new logo, "People and Science."

The Alzheimer's Association unites 160 organizations through its Coalition of Hope to raise awareness about the disease.

The film *The Notebook* is released (June).

Patti Davis's article " 'God Has a Plan,' My Dad Always Said" is published in *Newsweek* (June).

"As the Shadows Fell," an article on Nancy Reagan, is published in *Newsweek* (June).

Leeza Gibbons and Maria Shriver appear on the *Oprah Winfrey Show* to talk about their experiences as children of parents with Alzheimer's (July).

Sarah Sennott's "Ideas from Thin Air" about a video memory recorder is published in *Newsweek* (August).

Boston Legal television show featuring Denny Crane, a character with Alzheimer's, premieres (October).

Mary Carmichael's article "The Quest for Memory Drugs" about a hermaphroditic marine snail is published in *Newsweek* (December).

Maria Shriver's children's book *What's Happening to Grandpa?* is published.

Alive with Alzheimer's, by Cathy Stein Greenblat, is published.

2005

The Alzheimer's Association runs an ad campaign on how "Alzheimer's disease doesn't mean you forget how to . . ."

Mary Carmichael and Jennifer Barrett Ozol's "A Wrinkle in Time" about the science of aging is published in *Newsweek* (January).

James Bakalar and Anthony Komaroff's "The Aging Brain" is published in *Newsweek* (January).

"Artful Aging," by Karen Springen and Sam Seibert, is published *Newsweek* (January).

Angela Conrad's "Dependent on the Kindness of Strangers" is published in *Newsweek* (January).

The film *Aurora Borealis* is released (April).

"Avoiding Dementia: Fitness and Your Brain," by Steven Feske, is published in *Newsweek* (October).

Gray's Anatomy's Meredith struggles with her mother's Alzheimer's disease (October).

2006

David Sinclair and Anthony Komaroff's "Can We Slow Aging?" is published in *Newsweek* (December).

2007

The Good Life, written and directed by Steve Berra, featuring Harry Dean Stanton as a movie theater operator with Alzheimer's disease, plays at Sundance (January).

Alzheimer's from the Inside Out, by Richard Taylor, is published.

Time magazine publishes a special issue on the brain (January).

Carved in Sand: When Memory Fades in Mid-Life, by Cathryn Jakobson Ramin, is published.

Still Alice, a novel by Lisa Genova, is published.

The film *Away from Her* is released (May).

"Confronting Alzheimer's," by Barbara Kantrowitz and Karen Springen, is published in *Newsweek* (June).

Joshua Foer's article "Remember This: In the Archives of the Brain Our Lives Linger or Disappear" is published in *National Geographic* (November).

First StoryCorps Memory Loss Initiative story plays on *Morning Edition* (November).

The Art of Dementia Care, by Dan Kuhn and Jane Verity, is published.

2008

The film *Diminished Capacity* premieres at Sundance (January).

The Story of Forgetting, a novel by Stefan Merrill Block, is published.

Where Did I Leave My Glasses: The What, When, and Why of Normal Memory Loss, by Martha Weinman Lear, is published.

The Myth of Alzheimer's: What You Aren't Being Told About Today's Most Dreaded Diagnosis, by Peter Whitehouse and Danny George, is published.

Notes

Introduction

p. 2: The estimate of 11 to 16 million people with Alzheimer's disease by 2050 is cited by the Alzheimer's Association and comes from Liesi E. Hebert et al., "Alzheimer's Disease in the U.S. Population: Prevalence Estimates Using the 2000 Census," *Archives of Neurology* 60, no. 8 (2003): 1119–22.

p. 4: Viktor Frankl, *Man's Search for Meaning: An Introduction to Logotherapy*, trans. Ilse Lasch (Boston: Beacon Press, 1962). See also Frankl's *The Will to Meaning: Foundations and Applications of Logotherapy* (New York: World Publishing Company, 1969).

p. 4: The Alzheimer's Foundation of America and Forest Pharmaceuticals sponsored a survey conducted by Harris Interactive in 2006 that looked at stigma and reasons for delays in seeking diagnosis. The study, entitled "I CAN: Investigating Caregivers' Attitudes and Needs," is available at www.alzfdn.org.

p. 4: In 2006, the MetLife Foundation hired Harris Interactive to conduct a survey about U.S. attitudes toward Alzheimer's. Full results of the survey ("MetLife Foundation Alzheimer's Survey: What America Thinks") are available at www.metlife.org.

Part 1: Understanding Our Fears about Dementia

p. 7: Michael Ignatieff's novel *Scar Tissue* (New York: Farrar, Straus and Giroux, 1994), the source of the epigraph to the introduction, is the story of two brothers—one a writer and the other a doctor—and their very different struggles to cope with their mother's early-onset dementia. It's a complex and engaging tale that raises the emotional and physical challenges of dementia to a beautifully rendered symbolic level. This quotation is from page 10.

p. 7: The team of researchers who conducted the interviews about Alzheimer's disease included Shirley Huston-Findley and Kathryn Louis. Jim Herrington photographed most of those we interviewed, and Terry Caddell worked with me to create a short DVD based on the interviews, called *Talk Back Move Forward: 100 Years of Alzheimer's*. You can watch the DVD for free at www.aging.uwm.edu.

p. 10: Dr. Malaz Boustani presented data from the PRISM-PC survey at the Wisconsin Alzheimer's Institute conference in Madison, Wisconsin, on November 2, 2007. Eighty-one percent of the 335 older people surveyed said they feared a diagnosis of dementia would mean losing their driver's license. See also Malaz Boustani et al., "The PRISM-PC Questionnaire," *Alzheimer's and Dementia* 2, no. 3 (2006): S567.

p. 10: The Nietzsche quotation comes from maxim number 12 in "Maxims and Arrows" in *Twilight of the Idols,* first published in German in 1895; the translation comes from Viktor Frankl, *Man's Search for Meaning: An Introduction to Logotherapy,* trans. Ilse Lasch (Boston: Beacon Press, 1962), 84. The italics are mine.

Chapter 1: What Is (and Isn't) Memory?

p. 13: The epigraph to chapter 1 comes from the opening monologue of *Mnemonic* (London: Methuen Press, 1999), 4, a play by the European theater collaborative Complicite. I saw the performance in New York City at John Jay College in 2001.

p. 15: "Memories are not stored in any single location in the brain, as some researchers use to believe, nor are they distributed throughout the entire brain, as others contended. Different parts of the brain hold on to different aspects of an experience, which are in turn linked together by a special memory system hidden deep within the inner recesses of our brains" (Daniel Schacter, *Searching for Memory: The Brain, the Mind, and the Past* [New York: Basic Books, 1999], 9). See appendix B for Gülgün's shepherd's pie recipe.

p. 15: In a classic study, Lloyd R. Peterson and Margaret Jean Peterson determined that the duration of short-term memory is about 18 seconds (i.e., very short indeed!). They determined this by presenting research subjects with TRI-GRAMs (verbal materials) to remember while having them do some distracting task at the same time. They found that after about 18 seconds, pretty much everything in the subjects' short-term memory stores had been forgotten. This is still taught in most cognitive psych classes, although there are caveats, of course. Various mental operations that you can perform, such as "chunking" information into groups, will increase the duration of short-term memory ("Short-Term Retention of Individual Verbal Items," *Journal of Experimental Psychology* 58, no. 3 [1959]: 193–98).

p. 16: Maurice Halbwachs, *On Collective Memory,* ed. and trans. Lewis. A. Coser (Chicago: University of Chicago Press, 1992 [1941]), 38.

p. 16: There are long arguments about this point that I present fairly confidently and succinctly here. See David Manier's "Is Memory in the Brain? Remembering as Social Behavior," *Mind, Culture and Activity* 11, no. 4 (2004): 251–66, for a nuanced description of the disagreements between social theorists and those who believe that memory is strictly a matter of the brain and who tend to see "social memory" as interfering with encoding or retrieval.

p. 17: See appendix B for the cheesecake recipe.

p. 19: Peter Whitehouse and Danny George, *The Myth of Alzheimer's: The Story of a Disease, a Doctor, and a New Direction for Aging in the Twenty-first Century* (New York: St. Martin's Press, 2008), 36.

p. 19: See Daniel Schacter's *Searching for Memory.* For more on Camillo's Memory Theatre, see Francis Yates, *The Art of Memory* (Chicago: University of Chicago Press, 1966).

p. 20: Here are just a few examples of books on the history of memory: Mary Carruthers, *The Book of Memory: A Study of Memory in Medieval Culture* (New York: Cambridge University Press, 1992); Douwe Draaisma, *Metaphors of Memory: A History of Ideas about the Mind* (New York: Cambridge University Press, 2001); Paolo Rossi, *Logic and the Art of Memory: A Quest for a Universal Language,* trans. Steven Clucas (Chicago: University of Chicago Press, 2000); Paul Connerton, *How Societies Remember* (New

York: Cambridge University Press, 1989); David Gross, *Lost Time: On Remembering and Forgetting in Late Modern Culture* (Amherst: University of Massachusetts Press, 2000).

p. 20: Jacques Le Goff, *History and Memory,* trans. Elizabeth Claman and Steven Rendall (New York: Columbia University Press, 1992).

p. 20: Andre Leroi-Gourhan (*Gesture and Speech* [Cambridge, MA: MIT Press, 1993]) uses the term "ethnic" memory to refer to all human societies. Le Goff uses it only to refer to "the collective memory of people without writing" (*History and Memory,* 55).

p. 20: The story of Mnemosyne and Zeus can be found in Le Goff, *History and Memory,* 64.

p. 21: For more on the *libri memoriales,* see Le Goff, *History and Memory,* 71–72.

p. 21: Giulio Camillo Delminio was born about 1480 and died about 1544. His theater was born in response to theories of memory that organized human memory according to the planets. For more on the medieval European treatises on memory and on the "divine Camillo" as Francis Yates calls him, see Le Goff, *History and Memory,* 68–82, and Yates, *The Art of Memory.*

p. 22: For an academic framing of the issue of how photography changes our concept of memory, see Marianne Hirsch's *Family Frames: Photography, Narrative, and Post-Memory* (Cambridge, MA: Harvard University Press, 1997).

p. 22: See www.personalhistorians.org for more on the Association of Personal Historians.

p. 22: To learn more about Gordon Bell's MyLifeBits project, see his home page at http://research.microsoft.com/~GBell or Alex Wilkinson's article "Remember This? A Project to Record Everything We Do in Life," *New Yorker,* May 28, 2007, 38–44. Bell was also interviewed by Brooke Gladstone for National Public Radio's *On the Media* on January 5, 2007.

p. 23: To read more on video grave markers, see Jeffrey Zaslow, "Having a Say in Your Epitaph: The Challenge of High-Tech Tombstones," *Wall Street Journal,* April 7, 2005, sec. D, col. 2, 1.

p. 23: On the topic of the speed of contemporary culture, see, for example, Stephen Bertman's *HyperCulture: The Human Cost of Speed* (Westport, CT: Praeger, 1998) and his *Cultural Amnesia: America's Future and the Crisis of Memory* (Westport, CT: Praeger, 2000).

p. 23: The idea that postmodern society is akin to a state of schizophrenia comes from Gilles Deleuze and Félix Guattari's *Anti-Oedipus: Capitalism and Schizophrenia,* trans. Robert Hurley, Mark Seem, and Helen R. Lane (New York: Viking Press, 1977).

Chapter 2: The Danger of Stories

p. 25: The epigraph to chapter 2 comes from James's *The Principles of Psychology* (New York: Holt, 1890), 293–94.

p. 26: Stephen Hinshaw offers a thoughtful exploration of differences among stereotype, bias, discrimination, and stigma in his *The Mark of Shame: Stigma of Mental Illness and an Agenda for Change* (New York: Oxford University Press, 2007), 22–23.

p. 26: Erving Goffman, *Stigma: Notes on the Management of Spoiled Identity* (Englewood Cliffs, NJ: Prentice-Hall, 1963), 1–3.

p. 26: The "purpose" of stigma and fear of aging is addressed in "terror management theory" (TMT). The roots of TMT reach back to Ernest Becker's *The Birth and Death of Meaning* (New York: Free Press, 1971) and *The Denial of Death* (New York: Free Press, 1973). TMT was forged as a field of study by the work of Jeff Greenberg, Tom Pyszczynski, and Sheldon Solomon. See "The Causes and Consequences of a Need for Self-Esteem: A Terror Management Theory," in *Public and Private Self,* ed. Roy F. Baumeister (New York: Springer, 1986), 189–212, and Sheldon Solomon, Jeff Greenberg, and Tom Pyszczynski, "A Terror Management Theory of Social Behavior: The Psychological Functions of Self-Esteem and Cultural Worldviews," in vol. 24 of *Advances in Experimental Social Psychology,* ed. Mark P. Zanna (New York: Academic Press, 1991), 93–159.

p. 26: The "warm" but "incompetent" finding comes from Amy J. C. Cuddy, Michael Norton, and Susan Fiske, "This Old Stereotype: The Pervasiveness and Persistence of the Elderly Stereotype," *Journal of Social Issues* 61, no. 2 (2005): 267–85.

p. 27: Positive and negative stereotypes of older adults are listed in Mary Lee Hummert et al., "Stereotypes of the Elderly Held by Young, Middle-Aged and Elderly Adults," *Journal of Gerontology: Psychological Sciences* 49, no. 5 (1994): 240–49.

p. 27: For more on the association between the oldest old and the greater likelihood of negative stereotypes see Mary Lee Hummert, et al., "Judgments about Stereotypes of the Elderly: Attitudes, Age Associations, and Typicality Ratings of Young, Middle-Aged, and Elderly Adults," *Research on Aging* 17, no. 2 (1995): 165–89.

p. 27: Erdman Palmore, "The Ageism Survey: First Findings," *The Gerontologist* 41, no. 5 (2001): 572–75.

p. 27: Becca Levy et al., "Longevity Increased by Positive Self-Perceptions of Aging," *Journal of Personality and Social Psychology* 83, no. 2 (2002): 261–70.

p. 27: Institutional living might well contribute to cognitive decline by creating a culture of dependency and passivity. A study by Margeret M. Baltes and Hans Werner Wahl showed that long-term care staff members' interactions with residents encouraged dependent behaviors and inhibited independent behaviors ("Patterns of Communication in Old Age: The Dependence-Support and Independence-Ignore Script," *Health Communication* 8, no. 3 [1996]: 217–31). See also Jerry Avorn and Ellen Langer, "Induced Disability in Nursing Home Patients: A Controlled Trial," *Journal of the American Geriatrics Society* 20, no. 6 (1982): 297–300.

p. 27: Becca Levy and Ellen Langer, "Aging Free from Negative Stereotypes: Successful Memory in China and Among the American Deaf," *Journal of Personality and Social Psychology* 66, no. 6 (1994): 989–97.

p. 28: Levy's study on cognitive function and self-stereotype is "Improving Memory in Old Age through Implicit Self-Stereotyping," *Journal of Personality and Social Psychology* 71, no. 6 (1996): 1092–1107.

p. 28: For more on communication in nursing homes, see Mary Lee Hummert et al., "The Role of Age Stereotypes in Interpersonal Communication," in *Handbook of Communication and Aging Research,* 2nd ed., ed. Jon F. Nussbaum and Justine Coupland (Hillsdale, NJ: Lawrence Erlbaum, 2004), 91–115. See also Susan Kemper and Tamara Harden, "Experimentally Disentangling What Is Beneficial about Elderspeak from What Is Not," *Psychology and Aging* 14, no. 4 (199): 656–70.

p. 28: The survey, entitled "I CAN: Investigating Caregivers' Attitudes and Needs," was conducted by Harris Interactive in 2006. The study is available at www.alzfdn.org.

p. 29: For more on the health threats of stigma, see Brenda Major and Laurie T. O'Brien's "The Social Psychology of Stigma," *Annual Review of Psychology* 56, no. 1 (2005): 393–421.

p. 29: The study on elder attitudes toward aging based on television viewing is Margie Donlon, Ori Ashman, and Becca Levy, "Re-Vision of Older Television Characters: A Stereotype-Awareness Intervention," *Journal of Social Issues* 61, no. 2 (2005): 307–19.

p. 30: *The Simpsons* originally ran on Fox. This excerpt is taken from the episode "Lisa vs. Malibu Stacy," which first aired in February 1994.

Part 2: The Stories We Tell about Dementia in Popular Culture

p. 31: The epigraph to the introduction to part 2, a widely quoted phrase of Steven Jay Gould's, comes from his *Full House: The Spread of Excellence from Plato to Darwin* (New York: Three Rivers Press, 1997), 57.

p. 31: See Laurie Russell Hatch's "Gender and Ageism," *Generations* 29, no. 3 (2005): 19–24, for references to several studies about the low numbers and negative images of older adults on television.

p. 31: The 2 percent figure comes from the statement of Daniel Perry, executive director of the Alliance for Aging Research, before the Senate Special Committee on Aging, on May 19, 2003, reproduced in *Ageism in the Health Care System: Short Shrifting Seniors?* (Washington, DC: U.S. Government Printing Office, 2003). See also George Gerbner, Larry Gross, Nancy Signorielli, and Michael Morgan's "Aging with Television: Images on Television Drama and Conceptions of Social Reality," *Journal of Communication* 30, no. 1 (1980): 37.

p. 31: It's important to note the difference between stories told in a television show or film and the stories—character sketches really—found in commercials. A study by Darryl Miller, Teresita Levell, and Juliann Mazachek showed that positive images of older adults were prominent in television commercials between 1950 and 1990. See their "Stereotypes of the Elderly in U.S. Television Commercials from the 1950s to the 1990s," *International Journal of Aging and Human Development* 58, no. 4 (2004): 315–40. As efforts to capture the buying power of the aging baby boomers grow, commercials will likely continue to aim to inspire rather than offend older adults. Biases against older adults are reflected in the relative absence of images of them in mainstream media, in commercials aimed at younger people, and in the extreme (positive or negative) images of older adults in general.

p. 31: The number of images of older people in film is similar to that in television. See Martha M. Lauzen and David Dozier, "Maintaining the Double Standard: Portrayals of Age and Gender in Popular Films," *Sex Roles* 52, nos. 7/8 (2005): 437–46.

p. 31: The television executive's comment comes from Leo Bogart, *Over the Edge: How the Pursuit of Youth by Marketers and the Media Has Changed American Culture* (Chicago: Ivan R. Dee Publishing, 2005), 64.

p. 32: Ballenger explains how NIA founder Robert Butler argued that the government ought to fund the care of patients struggling with Alzheimer's as well as efforts to find a cure for it. But his eloquence about the need for scientific solutions undermined arguments for supporting care. Butler's vivid description of Alzheimer's disease as the new polio stuck in the minds of lawmakers, who were convinced that the cost of finding a cure would be less than the Medicare/Medicaid costs of care (*Self, Senility, and Alzheimer's Disease in Modern America*, 119).

Chapter 3: Memory Loss in the Mainstream

p. 35: The epigraph to chapter 3 comes from promotional material for *The Forgetting,* a 2004 PBS documentary on Alzheimer's.

p. 35: The figure of eight million viewers came from a personal phone interview I conducted with Boak in February 2007.

p. 35: The estimate of 100,000 books sold is a ballpark figure for both hardcover and paperback editions of the book from author David Shenk, which he gave me in a personal phone interview on April 7, 2007. Shenk said that it's hard to know exactly how many books have sold, as the author reports include promotional and review copies.

p. 36: I follow the definition of "epidemic" from Merriam-Webster Online (www.m-w.com/dictionary/epidemic).

p. 37: Madeleine Nash, "The New Science of Alzheimer's," *Time,* July 17, 2000; Claudia Kalb, Pat Wingert, Kate Grossman, Tara Weingarten, and Joan Raymond, "Coping with the Darkness," *Newsweek,* January 31, 2000, 52.

p. 38: Most recently, the Alzheimer's Association has been citing a study that puts the figure of early onset (cases under 65) at 10 percent of all cases, a significant jump from earlier estimates. What accounts for the jump are advances in brain imaging and earlier diagnosis of a condition called "mild cognitive impairment/probable Alzheimer's." For more on the history of this diagnosis, which is hotly debated, see Peter Whitehouse and Danny George's *The Myth of Alzheimer's: The Story of a Disease, a Doctor, and a New Direction for Aging in the Twenty-first Century* (New York: St. Martin's Press, 2008).

p. 38: The literal image of a house going dark is used in the film *Away from Her* (2007).

p. 38: For more on magazine coverage of dementia, see Juanne Clarke's "The Case of the Missing Person: Alzheimer's Disease in Mass Print Magazines, 1991–2001," *Health Communication* 19, no. 3 (2006): 269–76.

Chapter 4: Tightly Told Tragedies of Dementia

p. 40: The epigraph to chapter 4 comes from an episode of the *Oprah Winfrey Show* featuring Leeza Gibbons and Maria Shriver discussing the effect of Alzheimer's disease on their families, which aired on July 13, 2004. The episode also featured segments with Thomas DeBaggio, author of *Losing My Mind,* and Mike Henley, then 39 years old and living with early-onset Alzheimer's disease.

Chapter 5: Not So Tightly Tragic

p. 46: The epigraph to chapter 5 is a line spoken by Julie Christie, who plays Fiona, in the 2006 film *Away from Her.*

p. 46: Rocille and I talked in 2005 as part of a formal interview for the *Talk Back Move Forward* project.

p. 47: *The Forgetting: Alzheimer's, Portrait of an Epidemic* (New York: Doubleday, 2001), 252.

p. 47: I spoke with Naomi Boak by telephone in February 2006.

p. 47: Alice Munro, "The Bear Came over the Mountain," *New Yorker*, December 27, 1999, 110–26.

p. 48: I take my definition of "grace" from Merriam-Webster Online (www.m-w.com/dictionary/sanctified).

p. 49: Sean Axmaker calls *Away from Her* a poem on love and loss in "Poignant 'Away' Paints a Painful Picture of Loss," *Seattle Post-Intelligencer*, May 10, 2007.

Chapter 6: Not Tragic at All

p. 50: *50 First Dates*, which was released in 2004, was directed by Peter Segal and written by George Wing.

p. 51: Susan Sontag, *Illness as Metaphor* (New York: Farrar, Straus and Giroux, 1988), 79.

p. 51: For more on the first wave of amnesia films, see Robert Sklar as quoted in John Leland, "On Film as in Life, You Are What You Forget," *New York Times*, December 23, 2001, late edition, sec. 1, 1.

p. 51: Andy Seiler, "Studios Never Forget Amnesia," *USA Today*, June 19, 2002, sec. D, 3; Leland, "On Film as in Life"; Lev Grossman, "Amnesia the Beautiful," *Time*, March 29, 2004, 88; Terrence Rafferty, "The Last Word in Alienation: I Just Don't Remember," *New York Times*, November 2, 2003, late edition, sec. 2A, col. 1, 9.

p. 52: Rafferty, "The Last Word in Alienation."

p. 52: Catherine Myers of the Memory Disorders Project at Rutgers University–Newark addresses the limited number of cases of anterograde amnesia in Seiler's "Studios Never Forget Amnesia."

p. 53: Dr. Hovda's comments appear in Richard Pérez-Peña, "An Accurate Movie about Amnesia? Forget about It," *New York Times*, November 2, 2003, sec. 2A, col. 1, 28.

p. 53: Alzheimer's lack of cinematic flair is addressed in Pérez-Peña's "An Accurate Movie about Amnesia?"

p. 60: On April 21, 2008, the Alzheimer's Association announced its second group of celebrity champions and launched its second major paid advertising campaign. The 2008 celebrity champions included NFL football player Terrell Owens (chairman of the group), Anthony Anderson, Katie Armiger, Wayne Brady, Coach Frank Broyles, Dwight Clark, Emerson Drive, Hector Elizondo, Whiskey Falls, Leeza Gibbons, John Glover, Bryant Gumbel, Elisabeth Hasselbeck, Emma Mae Jacob, Matt Jenkins, Rafer Johnson, Lainie Kazan, Garry Marshall, Ronnie Marshall, Penny Marshall, Kathy Mattea, Terry Moran, Tony Plana, Ahmad Rashad, Jon Runyan, Rex Ryan, Molly Sims, April Taylor, and Anna Wilson.

Chapter 7: All of the Above

p. 61: The epigraph to chapter 7 comes from episode 2 of season 1 of *Boston Legal;* the episode aired October 10, 2004.

p. 66: Two episodes in the fourth season speak to Alzheimer's directly: "Mad about

You," which aired January 15, 2008, and "The Mighty Rogues," which aired April 15, 2008.

Part 3: Moving through Fear

p. 67: The epigraph to the introduction to part 3 can be found in vol. 7 of *The Journals and Miscellaneous Notebooks of Ralph Waldo Emerson,* ed. William Gilman et al. (Cambridge: Harvard University Press, 1960–), 241.

Chapter 8: StoryCorps and the Memory Loss Initiative

p. 71: The epigraph to chapter 8 comes from Jackson's StoryCorps interview, which took place in Los Angeles in 2007. It was broadcast on NPR's *Morning Edition* in November 2007.

p. 73: James Birren, Lisa Snyder, Lisa Gwyther, Henry Edmunds, and I made up the original advisory board for the Memory Loss Initiative in 2006–7.

p. 73: The survey on attitudes toward dementia was designed and tested by Susan McFadden and Melissa Lunsman. For a copy of the survey, contact McFadden@uwosh .edu. It was adapted for our purposes by my colleague at the University of Wisconsin–Milwaukee, Marie Savundranayagam, PhD. The surveys showed that the training increased the StoryCorps staff's comfort levels when they were interacting with a person with dementia. After training, the staff agreed more strongly that they felt "comfortable around people with Alzheimer's or related dementia (ADRD)," "comfortable touching people with ADRD," and "relaxed around people with ADRD." Second, StoryCorps training increased their understanding of how best to communicate with persons with dementia. After StoryCorps training, staff more strongly agreed with statements like "Difficult behaviors may be a form of communication for people with ADRD"; "I find it easy to communicate with persons with ADRD"; "Persons with ADRD enjoy being around other people"; and "Persons with ADRD still like to be part of a group." In addition, after training, the staff more strongly *disagreed* with the following statement: "It does not really matter to people with dementia how I talk to them."

The training also helped improve staff attitudes toward people with dementia. Story-Corps staff agreed more strongly with the following statements after training: "It is rewarding to work with people who have ADRD"; "I admire the coping skills of people with ADRD"; "Persons with dementia can still enjoy life a lot." Fourth, the MLI training helped research volunteers learn how to connect with and help people who have dementia. After training, staff agreed more strongly with the following: "I try to see the person behind the dementia"; "It is easy for me to emotionally connect with participants who have dementia"; "We can do a lot now to improve the lives of people with dementia"; and "I can make a difference in the lives of persons with dementia." Finally, staff became more knowledgeable about Alzheimer's disease and dementia through the training. After training, the staff more strongly *disagreed* with the statement that "I am not very familiar with ADRD."

p. 78: Zempsky expressed her hopes for the future of the MLI in a personal telephone interview with me on August 7, 2007.

p. 78: University of Wisconsin–Milwaukee CAC research associate Lorna Dilley conducted all MLI evaluation interviews.

p. 78: The full results of the StoryCorps MLI are heading toward publication, so I will not put all the details here. It will help readers of this book to know, however, that CAC researchers talked with 42 people with memory loss and 27 friends/family members within 10 days of the StoryCorps experience and with 20 friends/family members again within 3 months of the initial experience. Twenty-three people were in New York City, 16 in Chicago, eight in Milwaukee, and one in Richmond, Virginia.

p. 79: Mel was interviewed at the Lenox Hill Neighborhood House for its early memory loss program.

Chapter 9: Memory Bridge

p. 80: The epigraph to chapter 9 comes from a vignette about Annette, a former dancer diagnosed with Alzheimer's, and Jessica, her student-buddy, that can be found at www.memorybridge.org/classroom-page1.php.

p. 80: See appendix A for more information on these intergenerational programs.

p. 81: Jim Lambert, "Memory Bridge: The Foundation for Alzheimer's and Cultural Memory," www.imaginethisworldlearning.com/upload/PDFs/MemoryBridge_EdgeMag .pdf.

p. 81: Franchaun's buddy story can be found at www.memorybridge.org/class room-page2.php.

p. 82: Hall's description of a formal, sit-down dinner party comes from a conversation we had by phone in November 2007.

p. 82: Verde explained the kind of learning that takes place through the project to me during an in-person interview in February 2007.

p. 82: The story of the tracheostomy can be found at www.memorybridge.org/ classroom-page5.php.

p. 82: The story of the young man who had to cross rival gang territory to get to the program comes from "Gangbanger," which can be found at http://www.memorybridge .org/classroom-page6.php.

p. 83: The Memory Bridge student's story about Alice comes from www.memory bridge.org/classroom-page10.php.

p. 83: The quote "They seem to have more preconceived notions of care giving and aren't as open to the Memory Bridge experience" comes from a September 2007 phone interview with me.

p. 84: The quote "Now I see them" comes from my November 2007 phone inter-view with Hall.

p. 84: In 2007, the board of Memory Bridge also included Philip Stafford and June Kinoshita. Both were also founding board members in 2004.

p. 85: The comment about how people with early-onset dementia changed the students comes from my September 2007 interview with Cohen.

p. 85: The quote "People with dementia can remind us of aspects of our own humanity that *we* are forgetting" comes from an interview I conducted with Verde in February 2007.

p. 86: The vignette about Sam comes from www.memorybridge.org/classroom-page14.php.

Chapter 10: *To Whom I May Concern*

p. 87: *To Whom I May Concern,* from which the epigraph to chapter 10 is drawn, is an interactive theater project performed by individuals with Alzheimer's, mild cognitive impairment, or other related illnesses. The project has not, as of this date, been published. Author Maureen Matthews was kind enough to give me the manuscript version of both the 2006 and the 2007 plays.

p. 90: The remarks about the first performance of *To Whom I May Concern* come from phone interviews I conducted with Volkmer in July 2007 and with Matthews in August 2007.

p. 93: John Zeisel, founder of ARTZ, Artists for Alzheimer's, conducted the evaluations of *To Whom I May Concern.* In a telephone interview with me on September 27, 2007, Zeisel explained that the play had significantly increased awareness of dementia and reduced the stigma of dementia. The results of his evaluation had not been published by the time of this writing.

Chapter 11: Time*Slips* Creative Storytelling Project

p. 94: Gretchen, whose words are the source of the epigraph to chapter 11, is a Time*Slips* storyteller in Milwaukee, Wisconsin.

p. 98: Gülgün Kayim directed the Time*Slips* play staged in Oshkosh in 1997 and a second staged in Milwaukee in 2000. Paul Lucas and Gail Winar produced and Christopher Bayes directed the New York City–based Time*Slips* play in 2001.

p. 103: University of Wisconsin–Milwaukee's Center on Age and Community has conducted several research studies on the effect of the Time*Slips* storytelling method, including a study of 20 nursing homes that found, through surveys and extensive observation, that nursing home units in which Time*Slips* had been embedded had a significantly higher quantity of interactions between staff and residents with dementia and that those interactions were of a higher quality as well. The article on this study is forthcoming from *The Gerontologist.*

p. 103: "I Don't Look Like Him!" is a story that was told by a Time*Slips* storytelling group at Eastcastle Place in Milwaukee, Wisconsin, spring 2007.

Chapter 12: Songwriting Works

p. 104: The epigraph to chapter 12 can be found in the Songwriting Works annual report for 2005–6, available from Judith-Kate Friedman. B. C. was a participant in a Songwriting Works workshop at the Abramson Center for Jewish Life in Philadelphia, where Friedman was an artist in residence for 12 months.

p. 105: All quotes from Friedman in this chapter come from telephone interviews I conducted with her on November 22, 2006, and August 13, 2007.

p. 107: The "we start jamming" quotation comes from Dave Ford's "Judith-Kate

Friedman: Folksinger Stirs Seniors Creativity, They Write Their Own Songs of Hope," *San Francisco Chronicle,* July 26, 2002, WB–3.

p. 107: Friedman's discussion of her dream of recording the elders appears in Dave Ford's "Judith-Kate Friedman."

p. 108: Friedman told the story of the group's adjustment to 9/11 in one of my interviews with her; it is also recounted in Dave Ford's article.

p. 108: Rabbi Marder's comments about his mission come from a phone interview we had in September 2007.

p. 108: The quote "Everyone on staff knows *It's Hanukah Tonight*" comes from a phone interview I conducted with Allison in August 2007.

p. 109: Original words to *Peace Will Find a Way* are by elders on K2 and A2 at the Jewish Home of San Francisco and Judith-Kate Friedman. The music is by Judith-Kate Friedman, © 2003 Composing Together Works.

Chapter 13: Dance

p. 111: The source of the epigraph to chapter 13 is Brinkman Sustache's journal. She is choreographer for DanceWorks.

p. 111: All interviews with Katie Williams, Anna Liza Malone, and Dawn Adler, unless otherwise noted, were conducted during my September 24, 2007, visit to Luther Manor.

p. 114: For more on how anxiety and "self-esteem" have become medicalized, see Carl Elliot's *Better Than Well: American Medicine Meets the American Dream* (New York: W. W. Norton, 2003).

p. 114: I talked with Maria Genné by telephone on August 13, 2007.

p. 115: For more on the unique relationship between music and the brain, see Oliver Sacks's *Musicophilia: Tales of Music and the Brain* (New York: Knopf, 2007). See also the extensive research of Concetta M. Tomaino.

p. 115: Lerman's remarks here come from my telephone interview with her on October 8, 2007.

p. 116: Lerman's musings on memory also come from my telephone interview with her.

Chapter 14: The Visual Arts

p. 117: The epigraph to chapter 14 appears in Randy Kennedy's "The Pablo Picasso Alzheimer's Therapy," *New York Times,* October 30, 2005, sec. 2, col. 1, 1. Rosen took part in the Meet Me at MoMa program.

p. 119: Mollie Groshek shared the details of Oreda's art-making process with me in a personal letter, dated April 1, 2008.

p. 120: I interviewed John Zeisel by telephone on September 27, 2007.

p. 122: Janine Tursini made these comments about AFTA in a September 25, 2007, phone interview with me. All subsequent quotes by Tursini come from this interview.

p. 123: For more on the "Bushwick, Why Vote?" project, see my "Generations as Community: Elders Share the Arts and *Bushwick, Why Vote?*" written with Peggy Pettitt, in *Performing Democracy: International Perspectives on Urban Community-Based Performance,* ed. Tobin Nelhaus and Susan Haedicke (Ann Arbor: University of Michigan Press, 2000), 231–42.

p. 124: Rosen's and Brenton's quotations come from Randy Kennedy's "The Pablo Picasso Alzheimer's Therapy."

p. 125: Joann Loviglio, "Artist Documents Struggle with Alzheimer's," *Associated Press Online,* March 10, 2006.

p. 126: The article on Utermohlen that appeared on page 24 of the premier issue of *Eldr* in 2007 does not list an author.

Chapter 15: Duplex Planet

p. 127: The conversation among Kanslasky, Greenberger, and Brewer, the source of the epigraph to chapter 15, can be found in Greenberger's book *Duplex Planet: Everybody's Asking Who I Was* (Winchester, MA: Faber and Faber, 1994).

p. 127: The quote "I wanted others to know these people as I did" comes from an interview with Deborah Harper, president of Psychjourney, posted on www.psychjourney.com (http://psychjourney.libsyn.com/index.php?post_id=96195).

p. 128: The quote "the brain working faster than the mouth" also come from the interview with Harper.

p. 128: These conversations come from *Duplex Planet.*

p. 128: Greenberger's musings on fractured conversations come from a personal interview I conducted with him on October 23, 2006.

p. 129: These conversations are found in *Duplex Planet,* no. 163, 4 (note: it is not known if any of these people has memory loss).

p. 129: Greenberger talked about the misinterpretation of his work in my interview with him.

p. 129: The quote "like one of the few things I could do for them" comes from my interview with Greenberger.

p. 130: The quote "don't show me this" comes from my interview with Greenberger.

p. 131: The quote " 'I've heard that before, I'm bored' " comes from my interview with Greenberger.

p. 131: The quotes "I'm going to be dead" and " 'My Dad died' " come from my interview with Greenberger.

p. 132: Ann Powers, "Postcards from Planet Duplex," *New York Times,* March 5, 1993, 16.

p. 133: These conversations come from *Duplex Planet,* no. 147, 7; no. 147, 9; no. 105, inside cover; no. 163, 6; no. 163, 16.

Chapter 16: The Photography of Wing Young Huie

p. 134: The source of the epigraph to chapter 16 is an interview Huie conducted with Gil. Gil is the husband of Victoria (known as Vic), who has Alzheimer's.

p. 135: Huie described his process to me in a telephone interview on August 14, 2007.

Chapter 17: Autobiographies by People with Dementia

p. 145: The epigraph to chapter 17 comes from Stein's *Everybody's Autobiography* (New York: Random House, 1932), 68.

p. 145: Richard Taylor writes about how writing makes him feel normal in *Alzheimer's from the Inside Out* (Baltimore: Health Professions Press, 2007), 122.

p. 146: For more on how writing can relieve the stress of caregiving, see Howard Butcher, Kathleen Buckwalter, and Kathleen Coen's "Exasperations as Blessings: Meaning-Making and the Caregiving Experience," *Journal of Aging and Identity* 7, no. 2 (2002): 113–32.

p. 146: See appendix C for a full list of caregiver memoirs.

p. 146: Sue Miller, *The Story of My Father: A Memoir* (New York: Knopf, 2003), 40–41.

p. 147: Interviews with DeBaggio on *All Things Considered* aired December 22, 1999; March 16, 2000; July 11, 2000; and November 20, 2000. On May 20, 2005, Melissa Block interviewed Joyce DeBaggio about her husband.

p. 147: DeBaggio shared with me the story about the HBO film in an interview in November 2004.

p. 150: The quote "I write therefore I am" comes from Taylor, *Alzheimer's from the Inside Out*, xviii.

p. 150: The quotes "How will we know it is fixed?" and "From my perspective as a person living with the diagnosis" are from Taylor, *Alzheimer's from the Inside Out*, 11, 12.

p. 150: Peter Whitehouse and Danny George, *The Myth of Alzheimer's: The Story of a Disease, a Doctor, and a New Direction for Aging in the Twenty-first Century* (New York: St. Martin's Press, 2008), 6.

p. 150: The quote "much more a problem" can be found in Taylor, *Alzheimer's from the Inside Out*, 60.

p. 150: The quote "3,000-pound elephant" comes from Taylor, *Alzheimer's from the Inside Out*, 94.

p. 151: The quote "half-full / half-empty" appears in Taylor, *Alzheimer's from the Inside Out*, 105–6.

p. 151: The quote "Please understand, I am still here" is in Taylor, *Alzheimer's from the Inside Out*, 149.

p. 151: The quote " 'I'm a different Thou' " comes from Taylor, *Alzheimer's from the Inside Out*, 151.

p. 152: Robert Davis, *My Journey into Alzheimer's Disease* (Wheaton, IL: Tyndale House, 1989), 17.

p. 152: Diana Friel McGowin, *Living in the Labyrinth* (New York: Delacorte Press, 1993).

p. 152: Cary Henderson, *Partial View: An Alzheimer's Journal* (Dallas, TX: Southern Methodist University Press, 1998), 4.

p. 153: Taylor, *Alzheimer's from the Inside Out*, 31, 92, and 112.

Conclusion

p. 159: Dr. Malaz Boustani presented data from the PRISM-PC survey at the Wisconsin Alzheimer's Institute conference in Madison, Wisconsin, on November 2, 2007. Also see Malaz Boustani et al., "The PRISM-PC Questionnaire," *Alzheimer's and Dementia* 2, no. 3 (2006): S567.

p. 159: Increasingly, nursing homes are trying to serve the emotional and spiritual needs of residents as well as the physical and are aiming to preserve autonomy by responding to residents' choices. See www.pioneernetwork.net for more on the "culture change" movement in long-term care.

p. 160: Peter Whitehouse and Danny George. *The Myth of Alzheimer's: The Story of a Disease, a Doctor, and a New Direction for Aging in the Twenty-first Century* (New York: St. Martin's Press, 2008).

p. 161: Jeffrey Olick is the editor of *States of Memory: Continuities, Conflicts, and Transformations in National Retrospection* (Durham, NC: Duke University Press, 2003). He is also the author of *The Politics of Regret: On Collective Memory and Historical Responsibility* (New York: Routledge, 2007). Olick is in the process of editing another collection, *The Collective Memory Reader*, for Oxford University Press.

p. 162: The story about Umberto Eco can be found in Harald Weinrich's *Lethe: The Art and Critique of Forgetting*, trans. Steven Randall (Ithaca, NY: Cornell University Press, 2004), 12.

p. 162: Heiner Müller, *Explosion of a Memory: Writings by Heiner Müller* (New York: Performing Arts Journal Publications, 1989), 153.

p. 164: Gene Cohen, "Research on Creativity and Aging: The Positive Impact of the Arts on Health and Illness," *Generations* 30, no. 1 (Spring 2006): 7–15.

p. 164: There are a few studies on the effect of the arts on people with dementia, but all are small. See, for example, Clarissa Rentz and Jennifer Kinney's "Observed Well-Being among Individuals with Dementia: Memories in the Making, an Art Program, versus Other Structured Activity," *American Journal of Alzheimer's Disease and Other Dementias* 20, no. 4 (2005): 220–27.

p. 164: Thomas Fritsch et al., "Impact of Time*Slips*, a Creative Expression Intervention, on Nursing-Home Residents with Dementia and Their Professional Caregivers," submitted for publication to *The Gerontologist* in 2007.

p. 165: The statistic that those with more positive views of aging live 7.5 additional years comes from Becca Levy et al., "Longevity Increased by Positive Self-Perceptions of Aging," *Journal of Personality and Social Psychology* 83, no. 2 (2002): 261–70.

p. 168: Interview for *Talk Back Move Forward: 100 Years of Alzheimer's*, an 8-minute DVD I produced that emerged from a series of interviews I and my colleagues conducted and photographs we took in 2005–6. You can watch the DVD online for free at www.aging.uwm.edu. This quotation did not end up being included in the film.

Index

About the Author

Anne Davis Basting is the director of the Center on Age and Community and an associate professor in the Department of Theatre at the Peck School of the Arts, University of Wisconsin–Milwaukee, where she guides the applied arts and playwriting programs. Basting has written extensively on issues of aging and representation, including a book, *The Stages of Age: Performing Age in Contemporary American Culture* (University of Michigan Press, 1998). She has published numerous articles and essays across multiple disciplines in journals such as *Drama Review, American Theatre,* and *Journal of Aging Studies* and in anthologies such as *Figuring Age, Mental Wellness in Aging,* the *Handbook of the Humanities and Aging,* and *Aging and the Meaning of Time.* Basting is the recipient of a Rockefeller Fellowship, a Brookdale National Fellowship, and numerous major grants in support of her scholarly and creative endeavors. Her creative work includes nearly a dozen plays and public performances. Basting received her PhD in theater arts and dance from the University of Minnesota in 1995 and her master's in theater from University of Wisconsin–Madison in 1990. Basting continues to direct the Time*Slips* Creative Storytelling Project, which she founded in 1998. She is married to documentary filmmaker Brad Lichtenstein and has two children, Ben and Will.